PIONEER SPIRIT
Caring Heart
Healing Mission

Midland Health

~

Honoring the Past,
Creating the Future

Joe Tye

Pioneer Spirit, Caring Heart, Healing Mission

This is a work of fiction that is set five years in the future from the time it was written. Characters in the book might represent actual job titles at Midland Health but all names are fictitious. There are some programs and services mentioned, and some activities that are described in the story, that might or might not actually transpire; these are based on preliminary planning concepts being worked on at Midland Health when this book was written in mid-2015.

The following terms are trademarks of Values Coach Inc.: Invisible Architecture™, The Twelve Core Action Values™, The Self Empowerment Pledge™, The Pickle Challenge™, The Pickle Pledge™.

ISBN#: 1-887511-36-9
ISBN 13#: 978-1-887511-36-0

Self-publishing Partners: Studio 6 Sense LLC • studio6sense.com

CONTENTS

ACKNOWLEDGEMENTS

Over the years I have worked with many different hospitals. Midland Health, and the people who are at the heart of the organization, are truly exceptional. I especially want to acknowledge CEO Russell Meyers and Chief Operating Officer Bob Dent, whose vision for the future and commitment to the community and to their people were the genesis of this project. Kim Kincaid has been the indispensable organizer behind the scenes. Marcy Madrid has provided invaluable support both for this book and for the Culture of Ownership project. The executive leadership and middle management teams have been exemplary in their support for fostering a culture of ownership and promoting values training for their employees. Doctors Sari Nabulsi and Larry Wilson have helped to engage the medical staff, a vitally important but often overlooked element of culture change in healthcare. And a special note of appreciation and admiration for the 40 Spark Plugs who were in the inaugural class of Certified Values Coach Trainers (CVCT) at Midland Memorial Hospital.

Several hundred people were involved in focus group sessions and individual interviews as part of my research for the book, and while I greatly appreciate their participation, it's not possible to mention everyone by name. But I do want to thank Jimmy Patterson for the time he spent with me and for sharing his wonderful book chronicling the Midland story: *A History of Character*. Rosalind Redfern Grover, Barbara Tom Jowell, and Tevis Herd gave me several hours and a wealth of resources on the recent history of Midland Memorial Hospital and the effort behind the construction of the Scharbauer Tower with 100% community support. I also want to thank Conrad and Martie Coleman for their insights into the life and work of Dr. Viola Coleman.

As always, I am eternally grateful for the support of the Values Coach team, and especially for Michelle Arduser, Sandra Fancher, and my lovely wife Sally Tye. Lisa Peterson and her amazingly creative team at Studio 6 Sense gave us the design for this book, as well as *The Florence Prescription*, a copy of which is given to every Midland Health employee.

I also want to mention Mark and Bonnie Barnes, founders of the DAISY Award that is mentioned several times in this book, and which is visibly reflected on the DAISY wall at Midland Memorial Hospital. As we were working with Midland Health, Values Coach was also working with, and I was inspired by (and shamelessly stole ideas from) Susan Hall at The Guthrie Clinic, Deb Wilson at Kalispell Regional Healthcare, and Todd Linden at Grinnell Regional Medical Center (but in fairness I also let them steal ideas from Midland Health in return).

This book is dedicated to the fine men and women,
living and dead, who have worked to
make Midland Health what it is and what it will be.

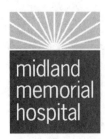

OUR MISSION

Leading healthcare for greater Midland.

OUR VISION

Midland will be the healthiest community in Texas.

OUR CORE VALUES

PIONEER SPIRIT...

- ⇥ We tell the truth and honor commitments.
- ⇥ We innovate and embrace change.
- ⇥ We are careful stewards of our resources.
- ⇥ We overcome problems without complaining.
- ⇥ We exceed quality and safety expectations through teamwork and partnerships.

CARING HEART...

- *We are West Texas friendly...* treating all people with kindness and respect.

- We care for the hearts and souls of our patients and visitors.

- We see the human being first and then the medical condition.

- We slow down and listen; true healing begins with empathy.

- We honor diversity and promote the dignity of each individual.

HEALING MISSION...

- We do our best to improve the health and well-being of our community.

- We are continuous learners.

- We create an environment that supports the healing process.

- We care for ourselves so we are able to care for others.

- We find joy in our work and have fun together.

FOREWORD

In the mid-1940's, a group of visionary Midlanders went to work building a Foundation that would develop the community's first full-service hospital. Seventy years down the road, I think they would marvel at the modern facility that stands as their legacy, and share our excitement about the future of healthcare in our growing community.

Throughout its history, Midland Memorial Hospital has experienced its share of challenges and triumphs, successes and setbacks. From the very beginning there has been one constant - the fundamental quality of the people who make up the organization. Employees and physicians, board members and philanthropists, all have shared a spirit of caring about each other and commitment to the community that is truly special and unique.

This book represents the culmination of a cultural initiative that recognizes the values and strengths of our people and builds upon them as we pursue a refreshed vision for the community's health. While technically a work of fiction, it captures the spirit that infuses this great organization and will power its future.

Under the umbrella of a broader organization we will call *Midland Health*, we are embracing our responsibility to see beyond the traditional confines of the hospital and lead all aspects of care delivery in Midland and the surrounding area. With the support of our generous community and the commitment of our people, our vision of building the healthiest community in Texas is undoubtedly within reach.

The amazing people of Midland Health are uniquely positioned to lead the transformation of our community's health in the years to come, and I consider myself truly privileged to be a part of this great organization. Thanks to Joe Tye and the team at Values Coach, Inc., for inspiring us to recognize the best of ourselves, and to build upon that strength for the good of those we serve.

Russell Meyers
President
Chief Executive Officer

PREFACE

After the Scharbauer Tower was opened at Midland Memorial Hospital in late 2012, patient satisfaction took a nosedive. That was because this beautiful new facility featured the most modern amenities and substantially increased patient expectations, but the actual patient experience was shaped by the same Invisible Architecture™ of values, culture, and attitude transferred over from the old facility. The widening gap between higher patient expectations and the same old experience resulted in reduced patient satisfaction. That was initially why Values Coach was retained by Midland Memorial Hospital – to help the hospital design an Invisible Architecture as beautiful and functional as the visible architecture of the new building.

Between the beginning of 2014 and the end of the year a great deal was accomplished. An initial cultural assessment survey was completed with a follow-up five months later; a new hospital values statement (that has been adopted as the title for this book) was finalized and approved; the Pickle Challenge resulted in heightened awareness of emotional negativity in the workplace and a nice donation to the employee assistance fund; The Self Empowerment Pledge has started to be woven into the cultural DNA of the organization; the course on The Twelve Core Action Values was launched; and a lot more.

The results have been amazing. From record low levels at the beginning of 2014, patient satisfaction was achieving record high levels by the end of the year. Clinical quality indicators were also hitting record highs. The second culture assessment survey reflected a dramatic improvement in cultural positivity at MMH, and one often heard words like "palpable" to describe the culture change throughout the organization. Patients and community residents are commenting on the changes, and it's even being noticed by hospitals in other Texas communities. MMH passed its accreditation survey with flying colors, with each of the surveyors commenting on how much more positive the culture was than in their previous visit. And the cultural productivity ROI has been estimated to be more than $7 million annually.

While these were all among the initial goals of the partnership between MMH and Values Coach, and we should all be proud of what's been accomplished, I'm even more inspired by stories I hear from individuals. I've spoken with people who have finally acted on a long-delayed dream of going back to school; started writing the book they've always said they were going to get around to writing "someday;" who have lost weight and gotten serious about getting out of debt; and who are taking what they've learned at the hospital home to share with their families. I even heard from one MMH employee that her daughter came home from school and said that her entire seventh grade class was taking The Pickle Pledge because the child of another MMH employee had shared it with the teacher.

Over the years Values Coach has worked with many organizations. The success at Midland Memorial Hospital is by far the most impressive we have ever seen. There are many reasons for this including the unmatched support of the senior leadership team; courageous commitment of managers throughout the organization to not allow this to be just another "program of the month;" a growing number of "spark plug" people throughout the organization who are really taking these things to heart (and not tolerating the cynics who want to rain on the parade); wholehearted participation by physician leaders; support from board members; and a healthy dose of West Texas friendly.

I am proud to consider myself a part of the MMH team and am excited to see where this journey of values and culture will lead in the years to come.

Joe Tye

PROLOGUE

Pioneer Spirit

The year was 1928. Dr. John Thomas had just finished installing the operating table in his surgical suite. He smiled to think that the newly opened 25-bed hospital on the top floor of the Thomas Building was, as far as he knew, the only hospital anywhere in the world that shared a building with oil companies, which had leased out all the lower floors. It's what you did on the frontier, where resources were scarce and people were resourceful. You made the most of what you had and you thought creatively to make up for what you didn't have.

It had been a long week with all the work that went into opening the new hospital. Dr. Thomas was ready to go home and have dinner with his family. But as he was putting the last of the supplies into the cabinet, he heard the sound of heavy boots come pounding up the stairs. The door flew open and a red-faced and out-of-breath man raced into the room. Dr. Thomas recognized him as one of the ranch hands at the O.B. Holt place, though he'd never met the man.

"Doc," the man wheezed, "we got an emergency out at the ranch. That young kid MacBride got bucked off his horse. His leg's broke pretty bad – you can see the bone sticking out."

The good doctor wrote off thoughts of an early dinner. "Is the break above the knee or below?"

The man blinked hard as if he was trying to visualize the boy's broken leg. "Below, I think. There was a lot of blood, you know, and I was in a hurry to get to you, so I didn't look too close. Payton and Mathis been holdin' him down, stoppin' the bleeding."

That was good news, thought Dr. Thomas. If the break was below the knee, at least it wasn't a fractured femur. And now he had a real surgical suite. He wouldn't have to operate on a kitchen table. "You got a wagon to bring the boy in?"

The ranch hand nodded. "They were getting' him bundled up when I left. I rode ahead hopin' to catch you before you closed up shop."

> THAT WAS THE SPIRIT ON THE FRONTIER. YOU DIDN'T NEED TO KNOW SOMEONE TO BE WILLING TO HELP THEM, JUST TO KNOW THAT THEY NEEDED HELP. AND THEN YOU DID WHATEVER NEEDED TO BE DONE.

Doc Thomas draped a sheet over the new surgical table and re-opened his black medical bag. "I'm going to need some help with this one. Can you run over to Mill Street and tell Josephine Guly - she's my nurse – to come on back. She'll be eating dinner but she won't mind you interrupting."

The ranch hand ran back out the door and pounded down the stairs. Dr. Thomas looked out the window and, as he saw the man running down the street, realized he hadn't asked his name. That's the way things were in Midland – that was the spirit on the frontier. You didn't need to know a man to be willing to help, just to know that he needed help.

It was a paradox he had often contemplated. People came to the frontier because they needed their independence, but they quickly learned that the only way they could survive on the frontier was to acknowledge their interdependence. He looked out the window again. At the edge of town he saw the wagon coming down Loraine Street. After checking again to make sure he'd laid out everything he would need, Dr. Thomas headed down the stairs. They would need help getting the boy out of the wagon and bringing him up the stairs. Perhaps in Dallas a doctor might think that such manual labor was beneath his dignity, but here in Midland you never heard the words "not my job." On the frontier, your job was doing whatever needed to be done.

Caring Heart

The year was 1976. Dr. Viola Coleman set her tray down on the table with a group of nurses. Though there was no celebration because she'd never said anything about it to anyone, today marked the 25th anniversary of her gaining privileges to practice medicine at Midland Memorial Hospital, just one year after the new 75-bed hospital had opened its doors. She smiled at the thought that when she'd first started working at MMH white people wouldn't sit with her in the cafeteria – not at first anyway. It had taken as much courage for the first white employee to come sit with her as it had taken for her to sit there alone on that first day. There was still work to be done, and probably always would be one way or another, but at least today there was no place for racial hatred in this place of healing.

Dr. Coleman had long ago lost track of how many babies she'd delivered, how many colds and sore throats she'd treated, how many broken bones she'd set, how many nights she'd gone without sleep caring for her patients. She never took account of the color of her patients' skin, and it was almost always the case that once a patient was in her care they never noticed that she was black. Only that she was a doctor, and that she cared.

"So tell me," she asked one of the nurses at the table, "how's our young man on the third floor doing?" They all knew that she was referring to Jimmy Madison, the kid who'd been admitted with a ruptured appendix and was now battling a pretty nasty infection.

"Well, Dr. Coleman," replied the redheaded nurse who'd just joined the hospital a few months earlier and was already proving to be an invaluable resource because of the experiences she'd had working at Parkland Hospital in Dallas, "he's doing okay. He can probably go home tomorrow or the next day. It's his Momma I'm most worried about."

Dr. Coleman gave her a sharp look. "What about his Momma?"

"Well, Jimmy wants to go to college and learn to be a veterinarian. He loves animals, you know, and he'd be good at it. But since his Daddy got hurt, his Momma says they can't afford college, that he's going to have to go work in the oil fields. I think his belly's healing but his heart is breaking."

Dr. Coleman shook her head. "Is she up there now? Jimmy's Momma?" The nurses all nodded. One of them said, "The bank gave her a few days off from her job so she could help take care of him. She's pretty much here all the time."

As Dr. Coleman finished her lunch she asked about the other patients on the floor. She asked each of the nurses about their families and they all made predictions about the outcome of the high school football game coming up that weekend. Then Dr. Coleman bussed her tray and walked up to the third floor.

Jimmy Madison's mother was in a chair by the window. The boy, who had just turned 18 and would soon be graduating from high school, was asleep. "Mrs. Madison, I'm Dr. Coleman. Jimmy's regular doctor is out of town for a few days and has asked if I could help look in on him. Your son's a fine young man and he's healing up real well."

Jenny Madison eyed Dr. Coleman suspiciously. It was a look she'd seen many, many times before. A look that questioned whether a woman – an African-American woman, and one who in certain parts of the community had a reputation for stirring up trouble - really could be a good doctor. "Mind if I join you for a minute?" Dr. Coleman asked as she pulled the other chair over to the window.

"It's a free country," Jimmy's mother replied, "I suppose you can sit wherever you want."

"I understand Jimmy wants to be a veterinarian. That's real good because Midland sure could use a good one."

Jimmy's mother shook her head and was about to say something but Dr. Coleman cut her off. "I know how expensive college is getting to be these days, and then there's vet school after that, so I imagine Jimmy's going to have to work to earn money for tuition." Dr. Coleman smiled and winked. "And to buy his Momma an occasional present for birthdays and Christmas and such." For the first time, Jenny Madison almost smiled. Dr. Coleman continued. "I've been speaking with the hospital administrator and he's telling me that we need to recruit more people. Town's growing, you know, and that means there are more sick people showing up at our door. Why don't I talk to him and see if we can't find Jimmy a job here at the hospital that pays the bills and still lets him earn his college degree. You know, an education is the one possession that no one can ever take away from you."

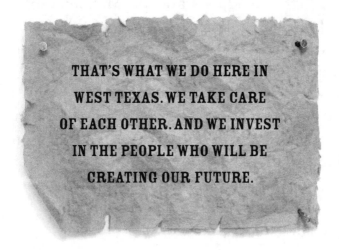

THAT'S WHAT WE DO HERE IN WEST TEXAS. WE TAKE CARE OF EACH OTHER. AND WE INVEST IN THE PEOPLE WHO WILL BE CREATING OUR FUTURE.

Dr. Coleman stood up and put a hand on Jenny Madison's shoulder. "Your boy's going to be a fine vet, and we're going to be proud to have him be a part of our hospital team. Don't you worry about a thing, Mrs. Madison, it will all work out just fine."

Jenny Madison swallowed hard and looked like she might cry. "Thank you," was all she could say.

"Oh, it's my pleasure. That's what we do here in West Texas. We take care of each other. And we invest in the people who will be creating our future."

Healing Mission

The year was 1986. Eight-year-old Jennie Scholander was trying to hold back the tears. The nightmares had returned. She didn't really know what acute lymphoblastic leukemia was – only that her doctors were trying hard to save her life, that she was tired all the time, and that because of the chemotherapy all her hair had fallen out. And now in her nightmares she found herself looking down upon a funeral – her funeral – from high above.

Jennie squeezed her eyes shut and willed herself to be strong and to not cry when the nurse she knew as Miss Rachel – who was her favorite nurse – came in to check on her. But then she thought of how sad it would be to never again run through the field behind her house, or to never climb another tree. And never to become a nurse like Miss Rachel. And the tears came again.

"What's the matter sweetheart? Does it hurt more today?" Miss Rachel sat on the edge of Jennie's bed and gently stroked her silky blonde hair. Jennie knew that she was Miss Rachel's favorite patient. She also knew that all of Miss Rachel's other patients believed the same thing.

"No, Miss Rachel," Jennie whimpered as she looked out the window. This hospital room had become her second home as she experienced the worst side-effects of the chemotherapy treatments. "It hurts the same as yesterday."

Miss Rachel stroked a tear from Jennie's cheek. "Then why are you so sad? Your Mom and Dad will be back as soon as your brother's football game is over."

Jennie could picture her big brother Matt out on the football field. He was in the tenth grade, already the team's star running back, and had told her confidentially that one day he would be a Dallas Cowboy. The sudden picture of her missing all of his games brought on a fresh bout of sobs. "The dreams have come back again, Miss Rachel. Worse than ever. I could see my family crying for me at my funeral." And now the tears flowed uncontrollably.

Miss Rachel scooted across the bed so she could wrap her arms around Jennie. She held her like that until the tears stopped. At last she said, "Jennie, you're going to walk again. You're going to run, you're going to skip rope, and you're going to ride your bike. And someday you are going to make a wonderful nurse – maybe even working right here at Midland Memorial Hospital. You're going to have to work very hard, and you're going to have to do some things that will hurt – maybe hurt a lot – to get your strength back. But we have the best doctors here. And you have me. We will never give up on you as long as you don't give up on yourself. And it's going to be a very long time before anyone is crying at your funeral. I promise you that. Okay?"

Miss Rachel lifted Jennie's chin with her forefinger. "Okay? Do we have a deal?"

Jennie wiped away a tear and sniffled. Then she smiled. "Yes, Miss Rachel. We have a deal."

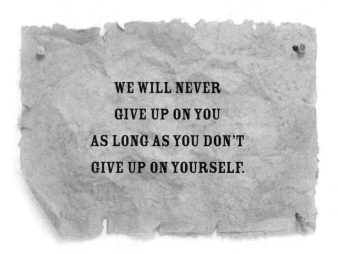

WE WILL NEVER
GIVE UP ON YOU
AS LONG AS YOU DON'T
GIVE UP ON YOURSELF.

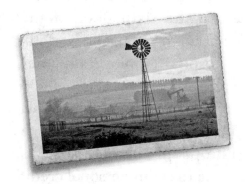

CHAPTER 1

The Market was abuzz with the news that a reporter from *The Wall Street Journal* was in town to write a story about how Midland Memorial Hospital had evolved from a small community hospital back in the 1950s into the Midland Health organization that was now being recognized as one of the most sophisticated healthcare organizations in the state, and how as a result the city of Midland had achieved a longstanding goal of being the healthiest community in Texas. Nobody noticed the two people sitting in the corner booth deep in conversation.

The man in the cowboy hat had the weathered face of someone who enjoyed working outside. If anyone could have seen him sitting there they would never have guessed that he had been one of the first physicians in West Texas and that through his hard work and personal investments he'd laid the foundation for what was now Midland Health. Dr. John Thomas seemed to be tracing an imaginary building across the table with his fingers. The woman sitting with him listened intently as he spoke.

Had anyone been able to see the woman in the long white lab coat they might have recognized her from the carved bust that was prominently displayed in the sixth floor of the hospital. They would have seen her laugh often, and periodically wave at one of the older hospital employees as they walked past, though no one ever waved back. When she'd first arrived in Midland, the hospital had welcomed Dr. Viola Coleman for her clinical skills but wouldn't welcome her to be in the cafeteria with the white people because she was black. Though she'd never been one to claim personal credit for her accomplishments, anyone familiar with the history of Midland knew that she was largely responsible for starting the movement that was reflected in the multicultural population now seen in The Market and in the larger Midland community.

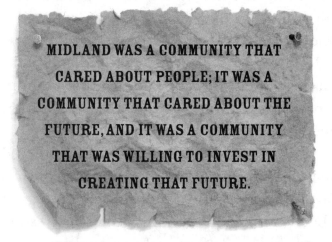

MIDLAND WAS A COMMUNITY THAT CARED ABOUT PEOPLE; IT WAS A COMMUNITY THAT CARED ABOUT THE FUTURE, AND IT WAS A COMMUNITY THAT WAS WILLING TO INVEST IN CREATING THAT FUTURE.

On this beautiful spring day in Midland the reporter from *The Wall Street Journal* wasn't the only person who would be wandering around the hospital asking questions. Though no one else would ever know it had happened, much less understand how it had happened, today two founding spirits who had helped to make Midland Memorial Hospital what it was had come back to see how their hospital was doing. Midland was a community that cared about people; it was a community that cared about the future, and it was a community that was willing to invest in creating that future – a future that included some of the finest healthcare services available anywhere.

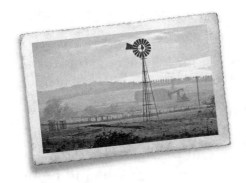

CHAPTER 2

"See the man over there talking on his cell phone?"
Dr. Viola Coleman tipped her head slightly in the
direction of the man in the blue blazer sitting
alone in a booth along the wall, although she could just as
well have stood on the table and hollered because nobody
other than Dr. Thomas could see her anyway. "He's *The Wall
Street Journal* reporter who specializes in healthcare stories. I
guess that *Texas Monthly* article about how Midland has just
been recognized as the healthiest community in Texas must
have gotten national attention, because that's what he's here
to write about."

They both watched the man making notes in his steno
pad. After a moment Coleman tapped the table and said,
"Well, since no one can see us we might as well go sit with
the man – hear what he has to say." John Thomas laughed
and stood up, then the two of them walked over to the booth
and sidled in, Viola taking the seat next to reporter Harold
Fillmore. He was taking notes as he spoke into the headset of
his cell phone. "It's a pretty big deal, actually," he was saying.

5

"To go from 37th five years ago to number one today took a lot of work by a lot of people. Yep – I've got appointments with about half a dozen people at Midland Health today. They were the lead agency on this."

Viola leaned in on her elbows and in a conspiratorial whisper said to her companion, "He's talking to his editor – trying to get him interested in the story."

The reporter scribbled something in his steno pad. "No, no – you're not listening to me, chief. This is a front page story, not a health column. It's not just about Midland being ranked as the healthiest community in Texas – oh, and by the way, one of only three Texas communities to be in the top ten percent nationally. What's happening in Midland is a metaphor for what's best about America – and for what needs to happen to get this nation back on the fast track. It's a story of leadership and teamwork, of courage and determination. If Midland – this little city-that-could out here amidst the prairies and oilfields of West Texas – can achieve what they have achieved, well, what can't be done?"

> WHAT'S HAPPENING IN MIDLAND IS A METAPHOR FOR WHAT'S BEST ABOUT AMERICA – AND FOR WHAT NEEDS TO HAPPEN TO GET THIS NATION BACK ON THE FAST TRACK. IT'S A STORY OF LEADERSHIP AND TEAMWORK, OF COURAGE AND DETERMINATION.

The reporter listened as his two invisible booth-mates strained to hear the voice on the other end of the phone. After a moment he said, "Well, you know the title is usually the last thing I write after the article has been finished, but I was thinking of using the three core values of Midland Health: *Pioneer Spirit, Caring Heart, Healing Mission.* It took all three of those things for this miracle of Midland to happen. What do you think?"

There was a long silence. Drs. Thomas and Coleman were almost as anxious as the reporter was to hear the response. At last they heard the editor's voice on the other end of the phone: "Okay, I like it – write a great article and you've got yourself a front page story." The reporter smiled and was about to respond when the editor cut him off. "So long as you meet the deadline. Got it?"

"Yeah, chief, I got it." The reporter smiled and looked out the window. A patient in a hospital gown was leaning on the arm of a hospital employee in a blue scrub shirt as the two of them slowly walked the labyrinth in the courtyard. The afternoon sun created the slightest shimmer of a halo around the pair. Fillmore scribbled a few more words into his notepad: *Change title of article to The Miracle of Midland.* He rested his chin on his palm and drummed his cheek with his fingers, deep in thought. There really was something special going on here. And he was going to write the story.

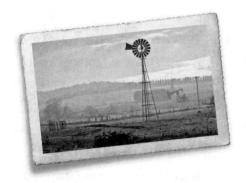

CHAPTER 3

Harold Fillmore looked at his watch. He still had another half-hour until his next appointment. He sipped his coffee and watched people walk by, scribbling notes in his journal.

"We can catch up with him later," Viola Coleman said. "I'd like to have a look around first." Two nurses passed by – one had a plate full of tacos and rice and the other had a big salad and an oversized cup of butterscotch pudding. "Hospital food sure has come a long way since the day I had my first meal here," Coleman said with a laugh, recalling all the old jokes about mystery meat and green Jell-O that regularly punctuated cafeteria conversations in her early years at Midland Memorial. "Come on, let's check it out."

They headed off in the direction of the serving stations but Dr. Thomas stopped them at a table where four physicians were carrying on an animated conversation. He leaned in and looked over the shoulder of a physician who had pulled up a digital x-ray image of a fractured femur on her tablet. As she described the magnitude of the injury and the course of subsequent surgery and physical therapy, she flipped through a progression of images showing various stages of the treatment process.

Dr. Thomas stood transfixed as he listened and watched images flash by on the physician's tablet. After a few minutes he turned to Dr. Coleman and said, "In my day that boy almost certainly would have died, either of the injury or of the subsequent infection. And if he'd survived, he most likely would have walked with a bad limp for the rest of his life. Now they can look right inside the leg, see what's wrong, go in and fix it, and next year he'll be back out on the football field. Amazing. No, not just amazing – it really is a miracle."

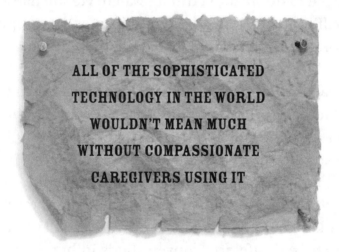

ALL OF THE SOPHISTICATED
TECHNOLOGY IN THE WORLD
WOULDN'T MEAN MUCH
WITHOUT COMPASSIONATE
CAREGIVERS USING IT

Dr. Coleman, who had also been viewing the images, nodded. "Yes, it really is miraculous what they can do now. But all of that sophisticated technology wouldn't mean much without compassionate caregivers using it. You could hear in that young doctor's voice that she wasn't just intellectually engaged with the medical technology – she's also emotionally engaged with a hurting young man." She watched a few more images go by, shook her head, and muttered softly, "Medical miracle – nothing else to call it." She took a slow deep breath, exhaled through pursed lips, then turned toward the serving area and said, "Let's go see what they're having for lunch."

The two physicians gawked at the virtual cornucopia that was the MMH Market. "My, my," Coleman said as they passed the sandwich station, the pizza bar, and the salad bar, "this looks more like a fancy restaurant than a hospital cafeteria. If the way to the heart really is through the stomach, Midland must have the happiest employees and patients in the world."

Thomas nodded in agreement. "I hope that people today don't take these things for granted. If we could send them back in time to my days, or even your days, and then let them come back, they would have a whole new appreciation for how comfortable life is in the 21st century." Coleman laughed while Thomas watched in amazement as a young man punched a button to make a chocolate milkshake for his little boy then said, "Shall we go back and see where all of this gourmet food is produced?"

They walked through the crowd back into the kitchen area. "This was always one of my favorite places to come," Coleman said as she admired the modern equipment. "Some of the hardest working, and too often under-appreciated, people in the hospital work in nutrition services. If they didn't show up for work one morning, this place would be in an uproar by ten o'clock."

John Thomas laughed and nodded in agreement. "If their not showing up meant no coffee," he said, "it wouldn't just be an uproar – there'd be fights in the hallways by ten o'clock!" They both laughed at this – then stopped when one of the cooks squinted in their direction, as if she'd actually heard something. Now the cook laughed, shook her head, and went back to her work. "Now I'm hearing things," the two heard her say. "No, darlin'," Dr. Thomas whispered, "you're not hearing things – you're just more perceptive than most people, that's all."

Before anyone else could say anything a man came out from the office near the back and shouted over the background noise, "Nice job, everyone. Monday's always a busy day, but between The Market and patient room service, today has been a monster day!" The kitchen the staff began to gather around the man whose nametag read Ted Fitzgerald, Director of Nutrition Services. "Who wants to lead us in today's promise?" he asked.

A young man that Fitzgerald recognized as having just joined the team the previous week shrugged and held up his hand. Fitzgerald acknowledged him and said, "Thank you Mike. Here, do you want to use my card?" He pulled a laminated card with The Self Empowerment Pledge from his clipboard and held it out to Mike.

"No sir, I think I've got it," Mike said, not looking very confident that he really did know it by heart. "I guess we'll see, huh." In the kitchen area the tradition was that one person would first recite that day's promise – either from memory or by reading one of the laminated Pledge cards that everyone was given during orientation – then lead the group in repeating it. Mike cleared his throat and closed his eyes for a second then said, "Monday's Promise is Responsibility. It says *I will take complete responsibility for my health, my happiness, my success, and my life and will not blame others for my problems or predicaments.*" Mike smiled, then blushed as the gathered group gave him an ovation. The sous-chef patted him on the shoulder. "Way to go, Mike – I'm proud of you."

After Mike had led the group in reciting the promise – which most of them knew by heart – Fitzgerald asked, "So does anyone have a story to share about today's promise?"

One of the longer-term employees raised her hand and was acknowledged. She crossed her arms and rocked slightly from side-to-side, which most of her coworkers knew she did when she was thinking, then said, "My son is going to school in North Carolina. At least that's what I thought he was doing. But he called me the other day and said he's dropped out because he's going to be playing in a rock band with some of the guys he's met out there. After he hung up I was getting all upset and worrying that he was going to get hooked on drugs and end up living under a bridge somewhere. Then I remembered today's promise and asked myself if this was a problem or a predicament. He's an adult now and he's going to find his way, and whether I agree with what he does or not, there's nothing I can do about it. So it's a predicament. I'm his mother so I'll always worry about him, of course, but it was pretty liberating to know that I could leave this predicament in God's hands."

Mike looked around the room and said, "I'm new here and still getting to know people, but I want to thank you all for welcoming me onto the team. And for sharing The Self Empowerment Pledge with me. I've shared it with my wife and we are both committed to keeping these seven promises. We say them every morning before we leave for work and again at dinnertime – and once more when we go to bed. We're taking better care of ourselves and we're getting out of debt. I can already tell that these seven promises will mark a turning point in our lives."

Fitzgerald smiled and gave Mike a thumb's up. "I can say the same thing, Mike. When I started doing a better job of keeping these promises at work I felt like I had to take them home and share them with my wife and kids. I might not be able to control what happens to me, but I can control what I do about it. It's my choice – I can complain about what's happening or I can empower myself to do something about it, and these seven promises have been helping me choose more wisely."

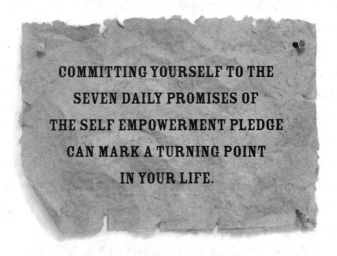

COMMITTING YOURSELF TO THE
SEVEN DAILY PROMISES OF
THE SELF EMPOWERMENT PLEDGE
CAN MARK A TURNING POINT
IN YOUR LIFE.

As the two time-traveling physicians watched everyone go back to work Dr. Thomas said, "I like that Responsibility Promise. Personal responsibility has always been a big part of the pioneer spirit of West Texas." Coleman nodded – she too had seen the power of taking complete responsibility in her own life. On the way out, they saw The Self Empowerment Pledge posted on one of the bulletin boards.

THE SELF EMPOWERMENT
PLEDGE

Seven Simple Promises That Will Change Your Life

**Monday's Promise:
Responsibility**

I will take complete responsibility for my health, my happiness, my success, and my life, and will not blame others for my problems or predicaments.

**Tuesday's Promise:
Accountability**

I will not allow low self-esteem, self-limiting beliefs, or the negativity of others to prevent me from achieving my authentic goals and from becoming the person I am meant to be.

**Wednesday's Promise:
Determination**

I will do the things I'm afraid to do, but which I know should be done. Sometimes this will mean asking for help to do that which I cannot do by myself.

**Thursday's Promise:
Contribution**

I will earn the help I need in advance by helping other people now, and repay the help I receive by serving others later.

**Friday's Promise:
Resilience**

I will face rejection and failure with courage, awareness, and perseverance, making these experiences the platform for future acceptance and success.

**Saturday's Promise:
Perspective**

Though I might not understand why adversity happens, by my conscious choice I will find strength, compassion, and grace through my trials.

Sunday's Promise: Faith

My faith and my gratitude for all that I have been blessed with will shine through in my attitudes and in my actions.

www.Pledge-Power.com

15

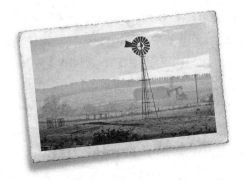

CHAPTER 4

"Mr. Fillmore?" The reporter looked up over the top of his reading glasses at a young woman in a blue business suit. "My name is Jennifer Scholander and I'll be making sure that you get to your appointments today."

"Hmm." Fillmore pulled the reading glasses down to the tip of his nose and held them in place with his index finger. "So, Jennifer, does that make you my babysitter or my parole officer?" He smiled and scratched his cheek, remembering some of the foreign assignments he'd had earlier in his career where the "tour guide" was really a secret police officer making sure that he didn't snoop around in corners where they didn't want him to be.

Jennifer laughed and blushed slightly. "Neither one – it's just that Midland Memorial Hospital is sort of spread out and we'd hate to have you get lost."

"Or stumble unannounced into the operating room?"

Jennifer smiled and nodded. "That too, I suppose. That wouldn't be too good, would it?"

"So," Fillmore said, "how long have you been at the hospital?"

Jennifer laughed. "You might say I've been here my entire life. I was born at Midland Memorial and was a patient here several times before I started working here. And in a way I was born here a second time when the team here saved my life. When I was eight years old they treated me for acute lymphoblastic leukemia. I lost all my hair but it grew back a different color that I like better than the original – a metaphor, I think, for the opportunity that can come from adversity."

Fillmore grimaced and looked at Jennifer over the top of his reading glasses. "So you're a survivor, huh?"

Jennifer laughed. "No sir, I'm not just a survivor – I'm a victor. I didn't just survive that illness; I grew stronger as a result of it. The things that most people complain about just roll off my back because of the perspective I gained from lying in a hospital bed at eight years old, wondering if I was going to live to be nine. Well, I obviously did. I went on to become an RN on our oncology unit, and now I'm the Director of Nursing Education for Midland Health."

Fillmore made a note in his steno pad. "Well, Jennifer Scholander, you just might make it into the article I'm working on – I'd like to hear more of your story if we get a chance." He pocketed his cell phone and steno pad and stood up. "So where are we off to, Jennifer?"

"We'll start with Human Resources. I'll take you the back way across the dock so you can catch a bit of West Texas warmth – I hear it's been cold and snowing in New York."

"That it has," Fillmore said as they walked out. "Let's walk slowly."

Halfway across the dock Fillmore did a double take at the carved wooden statue of a pickle that was guarding the door. "What's with the pickle?" he asked. "Didn't I see a banner with a big pickle back in the cafeteria?"

Jennifer laughed. "Yes you did. Around here we like to say that the pickle is a pretty big dill. As you are about to see for yourself." She opened the door and Fillmore stepped through – and found himself standing in front of a long glass wall with a giant picture of a pickle and the words "I've taken The Pickle Pledge" painted on the surface. Before he could say anything Jennifer said, "I think you're going to learn all about it in your meeting with our Vice President of Human Resources."

As they stepped into the HR department Fillmore saw another pickle banner on the back wall. This one said "MMH Pickle Challenge for Charity" at the top and had a thermometer-like scale on the side. He could see that the goal of The Pickle Challenge for Charity was to raise $20,000 and that that they were well over halfway there. "So what's this challenge?" he asked Jennifer.

Before she could answer a woman stepped out from her office and extended her right hand. "Hello, I'm Sarah Conlon, VP of Human Resources. You must be Mr. Fillmore from The Journal – which I read every morning with my coffee. And speaking of coffee, would you like a cup, or perhaps a bottle of water?" When Fillmore declined the offer Conlon said, "Why don't you both come into the conference room – I know you're on a pretty tight schedule."

When they'd settled in Fillmore said, "So, tell me about this thing you all have for pickles."

Conlon laughed then slid a laminated card across the desk. "This is The Pickle Pledge that you saw posted on our front wall. It says: *I will turn every complaint into either a blessing or a constructive suggestion.* And there's a footnote that says: *By taking The Pickle Pledge, I am promising myself that I will no longer waste my time and energy on blaming, complaining, and gossiping, nor will I commiserate with those who steal my energy with their blaming, complaining, and gossiping.*"

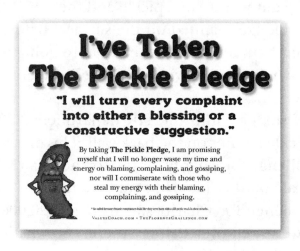

Fillmore picked up the card and read the text as Conlon continued. "We are working to make Midland Memorial Hospital – and ultimately the entire community of Midland, what we call a Pickle-Free Zone. PFZ for short. It's called The Pickle Pledge because people who are always complaining look like they've been sucking on a dill pickle, at least metaphorically speaking, and because a pickle is a nice fresh vegetable that has been soaked in vinegar, which is sort of what people with toxic negative attitudes feel like to be around. We are working to eradicate toxic emotional negativity from our organization. And it's working."

Fillmore was writing in his steno pad. "How do you know it's working?"

"Good question," Conlon replied. "Before I answer, a bit of history. The Pickle Pledge was introduced here something over five years ago. At the time I don't think anyone could have anticipated the way that it has taken hold in our organization. At first we were simply trying to help people become more aware of how complaining and criticizing, and talking about coworkers behind their backs, was literally like cultural poison. And not just for the organization – we wanted people to appreciate the harmful impact that toxic emotional negativity has on them personally – and on their families who catch the tail end of it after a long day at work."

She pointed to the pickle jar at the corner of her desk, which was decorated to look like something out of a Tom Sawyer and Huck Finn story. Looking closer, Fillmore saw that it was about half-full with coins. "The Pickle Challenge started when the staff of Midland Memorial was challenged by Values Coach – the company we've worked with on our culture of ownership project – to raise one-thousand dollars in quarters in a one week period by catching 4,000 individual incidents of whining, moaning, and complaining."

Fillmore's eyes jolted wide open. "Four-thousand?" he exclaimed.

Conlon laughed. "That was only two per employee. And between you and me, if we'd really been honest with ourselves we could have raised that thousand dollars in several hours. Well, we met that challenge. Values Coach matched it, as did an anonymous donor, and that money was donated to our employee assistance fund."

"I'm impressed," Fillmore said. "So what's with the pickle thermometer?"

"Well, most of the things that we complain about every day are really pretty petty when you look at what's going on around the world – or even in your own backyard. Someone came up with the idea that if we kept The Pickle Challenge going and kept on depositing quarters in these pickle jars whenever we caught ourselves complaining about something, we could keep adding to a fund that's there to help our colleagues who really do have something to complain about. So we set a goal of raising $20,000 in quarters to be donated to the fund – and as you saw, we are getting there."

Fillmore laughed. "If we fined everyone at *The Wall Street Journal* offices every time we caught them complaining about something we could fund the national debt!"

No one saw John Thomas and Viola Coleman standing in the corner. And nobody heard Thomas say, "I'll bet the same could be said about the guys working in the oil fields – or for any office building in downtown Houston for that matter."

Coleman nodded in agreement. "I've always believed that attitude is everything, and I'm glad to see they are finally doing something about it. Bad attitudes – what did she call it, toxic emotional negativity – have no place in a hospital."

Conlon leaned forward on her elbows. "While in the beginning this started out as a campaign to just get people to stop complaining so much, along the way something fascinating has happened. They are discovering that as they turn complaints into blessings and constructive suggestions instead of just whining about them, they have more mental space for positive emotions like love and wonder and gratitude. A lot of people have been gradually replacing habitual negative emotions with more positive and self-empowering emotions. The change has been palpable – and I don't think we'll ever go back to the way it was before."

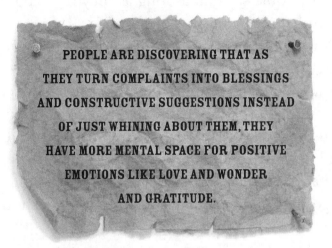

PEOPLE ARE DISCOVERING THAT AS THEY TURN COMPLAINTS INTO BLESSINGS AND CONSTRUCTIVE SUGGESTIONS INSTEAD OF JUST WHINING ABOUT THEM, THEY HAVE MORE MENTAL SPACE FOR POSITIVE EMOTIONS LIKE LOVE AND WONDER AND GRATITUDE.

Fillmore was scribbling in his steno pad as Conlon spoke. "The Pickle Challenge is one of the most important ways that we live our values. You've already heard about the three core values of Midland Health, right?" He nodded and she continued. "Our first core value is Pioneer Spirit. True pioneers don't complain about things – they do something about them. Our second core value is Caring Heart. How can you create a caring environment if you're surrounded with toxic emotional negativity? And our third core value is Healing Mission. I'm sure you've seen the research that shows negative emotions are both malignant and contagious. Part of our commitment to a healing mission is making sure that our people work in, and our patients are cared for in, a healing environment. And that begins with declaring this hospital to be a Pickle-Free Zone. And it continues with helping the people we serve to have the courage and strength to take care of their emotional health as well as their physical health."

Fillmore finished making a note then asked, "Don't you have some people say that as long as they're doing their job, their attitude is none of your business?"

Conlon shook her head. "Not anymore. Whether someone is coming in to apply for a job, coming down to file a grievance, or anything in between, the first thing they see on our wall out there is a very definitive statement that their attitude is our business, and that we are committed to finding solutions and not just complaining about problems."

Jennifer looked at her watch. "I'm sorry to interrupt, but they're going to be expecting us upstairs – we should probably think about wrapping up."

Fillmore nodded. "Just one more question. Have you lost some good workers because they didn't think their attitude was any of your business, or maybe had people not even apply when they saw that big pickle on your front door?"

"Actually, it's been the reverse. After the initial skepticism wore off and people realized that we were really serious about this, we've almost exclusively heard positive comments. In fact I've heard from quite a few people that they've taken the idea home with them and declared their homes to be pickle-free zones. And especially after the *Texas Monthly* article, we've had a big increase in the number of applications we get for every job opening. Just as we set a goal for Midland to be the healthiest community in Texas, we want Midland Memorial to be the most emotionally positive hospital in Texas."

"It does seem to be working," Fillmore said as he closed his journal.

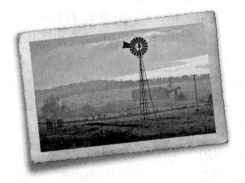

CHAPTER 5

T he two visitors from the past, not having to worry about such things as stairs and elevators, arrived at the sixth floor before Jennifer and Harold Fillmore did. Dr. Thomas nodded toward the bust of Viola Coleman that was mounted on a pillar outside the patient waiting area. "There are only two statues in this hospital, Viola. This one of you, and one downstairs of Florence Nightingale. You keep pretty good company. And you've left quite a legacy."

Coleman smiled. "I hope that my real legacy is in the people I encouraged to pursue their goals and to be the best they could be."

They heard the elevator bell behind them and saw Jennifer and Harold Fillmore step out. "This is the sixth floor," Jennifer was saying. "The long wing is for medical patients and the short wing is pediatrics. We're going to start with the long wing because the Clinical Manager is about to do unit orientation for new employees and we thought that would be a helpful thing for you to see."

Fillmore stopped at the bust of Viola Coleman. "Who's that?" he asked and looked quizzically at Jennifer.

Coleman looked at Dr. Thomas – who of course Jennifer and her guest could not see. "This should be interesting," she said with a smile.

Jennifer cleared her throat. "That's Dr. Viola Coleman. She was the first woman, and the first African-American, physician here at Midland Memorial Hospital. She's no longer living, but I guess when she was here she was a real force of nature. She had a big impact on the hospital, and also on the community. Later today our last stop will be the Coleman Clinic, which was named in her honor."

"A force of nature, eh?" Coleman laughed softly. "Honey, I'm just not sure about people remembering my legacy as being a force of nature. What's force of nature mean – that I was like a hurricane or a tornado wreaking havoc?"

"Sunshine is also a force of nature, Viola," Thomas said, "and look at all the good the sun does. And isn't that part of the calling of every caregiver – to be a force helping Mother Nature with the healing process?"

Coleman had already turned to follow Jennifer and the reporter. She looked back over her shoulder at Thomas and said, "Alright then, I guess I'll take that as a compliment."

At the teaming station they saw a small group standing in a semicircle around the Clinical Manager. Coleman surveyed the faces and the uniforms. "Hmm," she said, "registered nurses, patient care assistants, and a housekeeper. A hospital really is a small community, isn't it?"

Jennifer shook hands with the Clinical Manager then introduced her to Fillmore. "This is Andrea Jensen – she's recently been promoted into the role of Clinical Manager for the Medical Unit." They shook hands, then Jensen addressed the group. "Before we get started I want to introduce two guests. Some of you have already met Jennifer Scholander from Nursing Administration, and Mr. Fillmore is a reporter here from *The Wall Street Journal.* When we're done today he might want to ask some questions so please answer him honestly. Now, before I take you all on a tour of our unit I want to say a few things about my expectations of you, and what you can expect from me. First, you have all been asked to read and sign the Certificate of Commitment for The Florence Challenge, is that right?" She waited until everyone had nodded in assent.

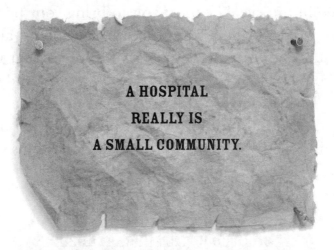

A HOSPITAL
REALLY IS
A SMALL COMMUNITY.

"Before you sign that I'm going to ask you to take a copy home with you and read it carefully. Sleep on it. If you're married talk to your spouse about it. Make sure that this is something you will commit to, because it outlines three of my most important expectations – and expectations of Midland Memorial Hospital – for our work together. I want to go over the three key elements of what you are committing yourself to. I'm passing around copies so that you will all be able to follow along with me. Okay?"

She looked every new employee in the eye before going on. "The first part of the commitment is being emotionally positive. I know you've all seen the pickle," and at this there was enthusiastic nodding of heads and a few comments to the effect that no one at Midland Memorial Hospital could miss seeing the pickle. "The Pickle Pledge is about being emotionally positive. Not just for our patients and for each other, but for you and your families as well. Life's just too short – or maybe too long – to waste it on toxic emotional negativity. So here's what I expect of you." She again looked each new employee in the eye. "I expect you to bring your best self to work every day. I expect you to treat our patients, and each other, with kindness and respect. And here's what you can expect from me: that I will treat you with dignity and respect, and that I will do my best to create an environment here where you can still be that best self when you go home to your families at the end of your shift. Any questions so far?"

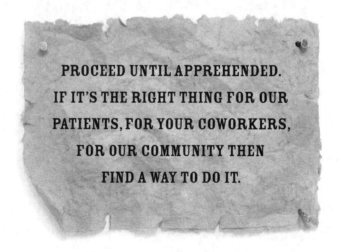

PROCEED UNTIL APPREHENDED.
IF IT'S THE RIGHT THING FOR OUR
PATIENTS, FOR YOUR COWORKERS,
FOR OUR COMMUNITY THEN
FIND A WAY TO DO IT.

There were none so she continued. "The second part of the commitment is to be self empowered. When you walked out of the room where you went through new employee orientation, do you remember seeing the big banner that said "Proceed Until Apprehended?'" She looked around again to make sure that everyone remembered having seen it. "There are organizations where a banner like that would be just words on the wall, but here at Midland Memorial Hospital we really mean it. If something needs to be done – if it's the right thing for our patients, for your coworkers, for our community – then find a way to do it. If you need my help, by all means ask me and I'll do what I can, but please never use me as an excuse for why you didn't do the right thing. And if you do what you thought was the right thing but I don't agree with it, we will have a friendly conversation about it, but I will not punish you for it. Are you all clear on that one?"

Heads nodded, but a bit more tentatively this time. "So let's talk about it. Someone give me an example of a situation where it would be the right thing to Proceed Until Apprehended."

After a few seconds of awkward silence the new housekeeper raised her hand and Jensen acknowledged her. "If someone wants you to close the shades in her room so she can sleep to go ahead and do it?"

Jensen nodded. "Good example. What if the patient asked for a cup of water?"

Before the housekeeper could respond one of the new nurses said, "Probably best to not Proceed Until Apprehended on that one in case the patient is on dietary restrictions."

The housekeeper smiled sheepishly. "I guess I've been apprehended, huh?"

"Actually," Jensen said, "this is a perfect example of why communication is so important, of why we need to act like a team. Over time you'll learn more and more about what you can proceed on and what you need to check with someone else on before you proceed. Any other examples?"

Another one of the new nurses raised a hand and said, "What to tell a patient who loses glasses or false teeth."

Jensen smiled. "You've worked on a medical unit before, haven't you?" Everyone laughed at this, including Scholander and Fillmore. "In a situation like that Proceed Until Apprehended means that anyone who works on this unit is authorized to reassure that patient that we will find the lost item or we will replace it. Of course, you have to use common sense. If someone says they've lost a suitcase full of hundred dollar bills, come talk to me before you proceed." This provoked even more laughter.

Looking down at the Certificate and then back at the faces in her group, Jensen said, "The third part is being fully engaged. Like I said, I will do everything I can to make this a great place to work, but I can't make you like working here. That is something you have to take personal responsibility for."

"That's today's promise!" exclaimed one of the new patient care assistants.

"Very good," Jensen replied, "I can tell already that you are going to fit right in on our unit." The PCA blushed at the acknowledgement. Before the manager could continue, Fillmore held his pen in the air indicating that he had a question. "Yes sir," she said nodding in his direction.

Fillmore pointed at the wall where The Pickle Pledge and The Self Empowerment Pledge were posted. "So I see these posters and I hear people saying the words, but how do you know they are really taking it to heart? I mean, lots of companies have slogans that they make their employees spout at company picnics and meetings – but are they real?"

"I can answer that," one of the new nurses said, and everyone – including Fillmore – looked at her with surprise. "One of the reasons I applied to work here is that a classmate of mine has been here for a couple of years and she kept telling me about these promises. I didn't really take her seriously but then," and the woman's eyes widened in mock surprise, "then she lost all this weight, you know. I mean, she lost like sixty pounds in a year. I asked her how she did it and she told me about The Self Empowerment Pledge, how once she started to be responsible, accountable, and determined she started to change her life. And not just her weight – she's getting out of debt and she's working out and she's a lot happier at home. And I thought, man – I want to work for a place that cares enough to share these things with employees. So here I am."

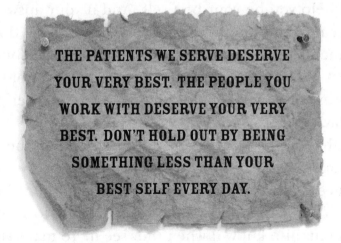

THE PATIENTS WE SERVE DESERVE YOUR VERY BEST. THE PEOPLE YOU WORK WITH DESERVE YOUR VERY BEST. DON'T HOLD OUT BY BEING SOMETHING LESS THAN YOUR BEST SELF EVERY DAY.

"We hear lots of stories like that," Jensen said. "At first people might just be saying the words, but after while the words sink in and they start to make changes. I know I have." Now she looked over to a woman who'd been standing next to her, but who hadn't yet spoken. "I want to introduce you to my friend Martha Bannock. She's a two-time DAISY Award winner." She saw Fillmore cock his head so she added, "DAISY Awards are given in recognition of nursing excellence. You might have seen the DAISY wall down by the cafeteria."

"I'll show it to you when we go back down for lunch," Jennifer whispered. Jensen nodded to Martha and said, "Can you share a few comments about what the DAISY Award means to you?"

"You bet," Martha replied. "I want to emphasize two terms you've already heard: best self and kindness. One of the things I really took away from the course on The Twelve Core Action Values is the Direction Deflection Question. It simply means that before you say or do something you stop and ask yourself whether whatever it is you're about to do or say will help you be your best self. And if your answer is no, then the next question is what would your best self do or say? The patients we serve all deserve your very best. The people you work with all deserve your very best. Don't hold out on us by bringing something less than the very best self to work every day."

Martha stopped to gauge the reactions of the people to whom she was speaking. Pleased with what she saw, she continued. "We all know kindness when we see it but on a fast-paced unit like ours, sometimes it's easy to forget that our patients also know it when they see it. To make sure that never happens to me, I play a little game with myself. Before

I go into a patient's room, or have a difficult conversation with a coworker, I imagine Florence Nightingale standing at my shoulder. It might sound silly, since she's been dead for a long time, but that simple thing – just imagining her standing there – helps me to always act as my best self and to treat others with the kindness they deserve."

Viola Coleman looked at John Thomas. "That doesn't sound silly to me, does it to you? Everybody needs heroes and role models. So what if they don't happen to be alive anymore?"

"Viola," he replied, "that's why your face is the first thing people see when they come onto this unit."

> BEFORE YOU GO INTO A PATIENT'S ROOM, OR HAVE A DIFFICULT CONVERSATION WITH A COWORKER, IMAGINE FLORENCE NIGHTINGALE STANDING AT YOUR SHOULDER TELLING YOU THE BEST THING TO DO IN THAT SITUATION.

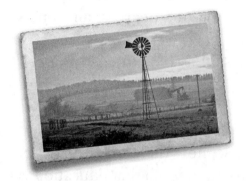

CHAPTER 6

After leaving the Medical Unit, Jennifer led Harold Fillmore towards Pediatrics. Dr. Thomas and Dr. Coleman followed unnoticed. On the wall just inside the door was a banner that read:

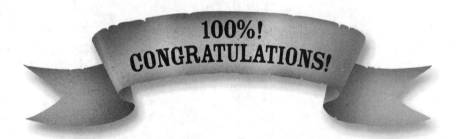

100%!
CONGRATULATIONS!

They were greeted by Randy Murphy, the Clinical Manager for Pediatrics. After introductions were made Fillmore asked, "What's the 100% for – customer satisfaction?"

"Well," replied Murphy, "first of all we don't call the little ones in our care customers – they are our patients. We treat them as we would our own children. We're here to serve them, not to sell them something. And yes we do strive for 100% satisfaction, but that's not what this banner is for. Three of our registered nurses just graduated with their BSN degrees and we are now 100% at least baccalaureate degree prepared. And several of our nurses have masters degrees, and one's working on a DNP degree."

"Very impressive," Fillmore said as he extracted the cell phone from his sports coat pocket. "Mind if I take a picture of your banner?"

As Fillmore was taking his picture, Dr. Coleman turned to Dr. Thomas who was, of course, not visible to anyone else, and said, "I always would tell young people that education is one thing no one can ever take away from you. I am so glad to see the emphasis they are putting on encouraging people to pursue learning."

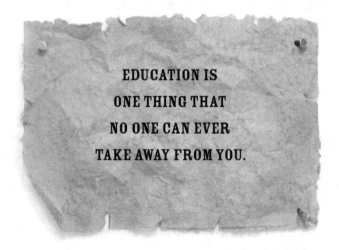

EDUCATION IS
ONE THING THAT
NO ONE CAN EVER
TAKE AWAY FROM YOU.

At that moment they saw a little girl with taffy-pull pigtails and a Texas-sized smile on her face coming down the hallway driving a kid-sized motorized vehicle. "And I'm glad to see that they let these little people drive their little cars around the unit," said Coleman. "I've always believed that it's important to get up and get moving as soon as you can after you've been knocked down." Then she laughed and said, "but it doesn't look like much could keep this young lady down for long."

"Hi Munchkin, how are you feeling today?" Murphy asked as he leaned over to give the little girl a gentle pat on the head. "You look a lot better than you did yesterday."

"I'm racing the boys," the little girl replied, then added, "but you can't see them because their cars are invisible."

"We all need invisible friends, don't we?" Murphy replied. "Do you remember Jennifer, sweetheart? She was up here yesterday." The little girl nodded. "And this is Mr. Fillmore. He is writing a story about our hospital and our town."

"Who's she?" said the little girl, pointing towards a Viola Coleman that the adults around her could not see. At this, Dr. Coleman leaned over with her hands on her knees and said, "Honey, I'm another invisible friend here to make sure they're taking good care of you. So we'll just keep that a little secret between you and me, okay?"

The little girl nodded emphatically then looked up at Fillmore. "Can I be in your story?"

"Well, young lady, I think that just might be possible. I'll tell you what – when we're done with all the grownup talk can I ask you some questions?"

The little girl laughed and squealed with delight. "Of course you can – didn't you read the sign?"

"What sign," Fillmore replied but she had already pressed on the accelerator of her little electric car and was buzzing down the corridor. "What sign?" he asked again, this time looking at Randy Murphy.

"I'll show you," Murphy said and guided them back to the teaming station. There he pointed to a sign next to the white board that read:

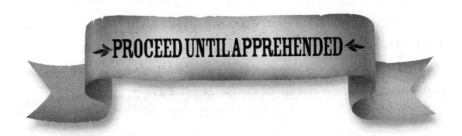

→ PROCEED UNTIL APPREHENDED ←

"Those are three words you tend to hear a lot around here," Murphy said with a smile.

"Even from your littlest patients, evidently," Fillmore replied.

Looking down the corridor Murphy saw a man in a long white lab coat and waved for him to come join the group. When the physician arrived at the teaming station Murphy introduced him. "This is Dr. Eric Martin. A big part of the story of the Midland Health cultural transformation has been the positive role played by the medical staff, and Eric has been a leader in the effort."

The little girl with the taffy-pull pigtails waved as she again drove the other way past the teaming station. "She is a brave little girl," Murphy said. "These kids inspire us as much as we help them." Murphy gave her a thumbs up as she scooted by then said, "Dr. Martin, this is Harold Fillmore from *The Wall Street Journal*. He's here to write a story about how Midland became the healthiest community in Texas – and of course include how the medical staff played a big part in the achievement."

The two men shook hands and Fillmore said, "So, tell me about it – how did this transformation take place?" He pulled out his steno pad and a pen. When Murphy looked on with surprise Fillmore smiled and said, "I'm old school – I still like the feel of a pen gliding across the page."

Dr. Martin laughed and said, "Me too!" and pulled a pen and journal from the pocket of his lab coat. "I'm really proud of the way my colleagues have embraced this culture of ownership. We've seen how it provides better clinical care, happier patients, and made it a better place to work. As physicians, we like to see structure – we sometimes have a hard time dealing with abstractions like corporate culture. But we all got, and most of us have read, a book called *The Florence Prescription* that describes a structured approach by defining the essential characteristics of a culture of ownership." Martin pointed to a small poster on the wall. "This structure helped us go from an 'I'll know it when I see it' approach to defining a great culture to helping us know just what to look for."

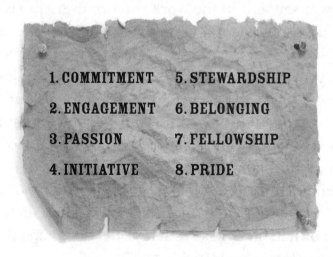

1. COMMITMENT 5. STEWARDSHIP

2. ENGAGEMENT 6. BELONGING

3. PASSION 7. FELLOWSHIP

4. INITIATIVE 8. PRIDE

As Fillmore again took out his cell phone to take a picture of the poster Dr. Martin continued. "We started with the first three – making sure that we were all committed to our mission, engaged with our patients and with each other, and passionate about the work we did. We saw those three things as being a prerequisite to the next two – initiative and stewardship; people who are thinking like owners take the initiative and do what needs to be done – they proceed until apprehended – and they take care to be good stewards of the organization's resources. And with a culture of ownership we want everyone to have a sense of belonging, so we are very open about sharing information, and to have a spirit of fellowship, so we embrace everyone as a key member of our team."

Martin tapped the last characteristic with his index finger. "When you get the first seven characteristics right then pride is the culmination, the icing on the cake. Up here we talk about the four cornerstones of pride. The first cornerstone is pride in yourself and in the work you do. Every job is important and we expect people to be proud of what they do and how they do it. The second is pride in your profession; we want everyone on our unit – from housekeeper to doctorate level nurse – to see themselves as a professional. And finally, we want everyone to be proud of our Pediatrics unit and be proud to say that they work at Midland Memorial Hospital."

Fillmore finished making a note, then looked at the unit's decorated pickle jar. "I apologize, guys, but as a reporter I am obligated to ask the tough questions. If you have such a great culture of ownership and so much pride, how come there are so many quarters in your pickle jar?"

Murphy laughed. "When The Pickle Challenge first started most of us thought we didn't need it because we were all pretty positive up here. But we're team players, so we went along with it. And I think we were all a bit shocked to see how fast the whine fines – that's what we called the quarters we had to deposit if we were caught whining – at how fast they piled up."

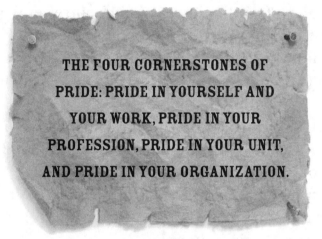

THE FOUR CORNERSTONES OF PRIDE: PRIDE IN YOURSELF AND YOUR WORK, PRIDE IN YOUR PROFESSION, PRIDE IN YOUR UNIT, AND PRIDE IN YOUR ORGANIZATION.

Now Dr. Martin laughed. "The word shocked might be an understatement – had we caught all of them, I think we might have filled up that pickle jar every day."

"But what started to happen," Murphy continued, "was that we started changing our habits. We really did start to see blessings and look for constructive suggestions instead of just complaining about things. We smiled more, we said 'thank you' more, and we stopped wasting our time and emotional energy on toxic emotional negativity."

Fillmore pulled out his cell phone and snapped a picture of the pickle jar. "So if you've broken all those nasty old complaining habits and it's so much more positive up here, then why does your pickle jar have so many coins in it?"

"Well," Murphy replied, "we want to do our part to help the hospital reach the goal, so we added a category. So now whenever I or anyone else sees someone turning a complaint into a blessing or a constructive suggestion they can take a quarter out of the manager's discretionary fund," and here he pointed to a bowl half-full of quarters on the counter, "and put it in the jar. That way we are still doing our part for the challenge, and continuing to remind ourselves that we want this to be the most positive kid's unit in the world."

The little girl in the tiny motor car drove past again. "Bet you can't apprehend me!" she yelled as she maneuvered the car into a patient room.

"Well," Murphy said as he put a hand on Dr. Martin's shoulder, "it looks like we have some apprehending to do before we can give Traci her medication."

The two men were headed for the little girl's room when the tiny car emerged again and took a sharp right, leaving Murphy and Martin in its wake.

"Did they have cars like that when you were here as a kid?" Fillmore asked Jennifer. "Are you kidding?" she replied. "When I was a kid we raced around in hijacked wheelchairs powered by our scrawny little muscles."

Dr. Thomas laughed and said, "You know, Viola, I wish I would have thought of this. Back in my day we could have had wooden horses for the kids to ride."

Dr. Coleman smiled as she watched the little girl again elude the nurse and the physician who were pretending to be trying to catch her. "It's good to see that old saying that laughter is the best medicine actually being put into practice here in the hospital."

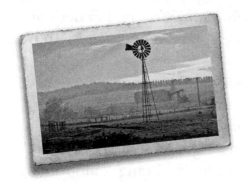

CHAPTER 7

J ennifer led Fillmore out of the elevator toward the long corridor by the conference center. When he saw the wall he stopped, did a double take, and just stood there with his mouth open. Jennifer smiled. Everyone reacted this way. She waited for him to say something. Finally he said, "What is this?"

"That's our commitment wall – well, one of them," she replied. "What you are seeing is – at last count – some of the 2,459 signed Certificates of Commitment for The Florence Challenge that Andrea Jensen talked about when we were on the 6th floor medical unit. You'll see these certificates posted on walls like this all around Midland Health. If you look more closely you'll see that many of them also have the employee's photo next to their signature. There's one for almost every Midland Health employee."

Fillmore stepped closer to the wall and began reading the text on one of the certificates. "So employees are required to sign one of these?"

"No, it's voluntary." Jennifer waved an arm along the wall. "But we find that people who are enthusiastic about making the commitment are most likely to have a great experience being part of our team. And we're at pretty close to 100% participation."

Fillmore took out his cell phone and snapped a close-up of one of the signed certificates, then stepped back and took several pictures of the entire wall. "So," he asked, "just what are people committing themselves to when they sign one of these?"

"Three things," Jennifer replied. "Being emotionally positive, being self empowered, and being fully engaged. We believe that those are the three essential ingredients of a great culture – of being both a great place to work and a great place to receive care. When the survey team came to Midland from the Great Place to Work Institute, I think they were more impressed by this wall than any other single thing they saw."

Jennifer stepped closer to the wall and placed a finger on the first line of one of the certificates. "The first thing people are committing themselves to by signing a certificate is being emotionally positive. We've found that the most powerful and effective tool for encouraging emotional health and positive attitudes is The Pickle Pledge – that promise you saw when we were at the Human Resources department. It really is a life-changing shift of consciousness when instead of complaining about what's wrong with our lives, we learn to see the blessings and look for ways to make things better."

Fillmore had taken out his steno pad and was making notes. Jennifer continued. "What many of us have found is that the greatest benefit of taking The Pickle Pledge isn't just how it changes our attitudes at work, as important as that is. The real benefit is the way it can change the family dynamic at home. When I shared this with my kids – I have a girl 12 and a boy 9 – they took to it almost immediately. Instead of whining about having to get up and go to school, they'll talk about a beautiful sunrise, or how much they're looking forward to the football game on Friday night. And my husband – God love him, he's a good man, but he used to complain about everything. He still backslides on occasion, but he's down to just a few quarters a day."

Fillmore laughed and shook his head. "Please don't tell my wife that the Pickle Challenge can also be taken home – she'd have my life savings in the pickle jar in about six weeks!"

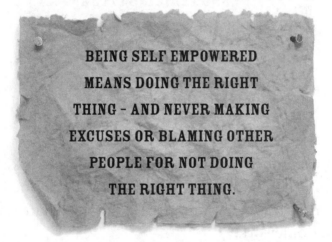

BEING SELF EMPOWERED
MEANS DOING THE RIGHT
THING - AND NEVER MAKING
EXCUSES OR BLAMING OTHER
PEOPLE FOR NOT DOING
THE RIGHT THING.

Jennifer laughed, then placed a finger on the second line of the certificate. "Being self empowered means doing the right thing – and never making excuses or blaming other people for not doing the right thing. As you've already seen, something you'll hear a lot around here are the words 'Proceed Until Apprehended.' That doesn't mean you can be a loose cannon – it means that if it's the right thing to do for a patient, for a coworker, or for our community, you find a way to get it done. You proceed until apprehended."

Jennifer gave her wristband a gentle tug. "You'll also see a lot of people around here wearing these. In fact, I'm sure that someone will give you a set before you leave. There's a different color wristband for each one of the seven promises of The Self Empowerment Pledge. Today I'm wearing one for Monday's Promise on Responsibility."

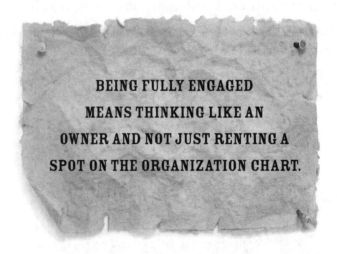

BEING FULLY ENGAGED MEANS THINKING LIKE AN OWNER AND NOT JUST RENTING A SPOT ON THE ORGANIZATION CHART.

"And what does that promise say?" Fillmore asked with a mischievous smile, then crossed his arms and tapped his foot like a school teacher waiting to see if a student really had done the homework.

Jennifer returned the smile. "By now most of us have the promises pretty much memorized. Today's promise says: I will take complete responsibility for my health, my happiness, my success, and my life and will not blame others for my problems or predicaments."

"Very good," Fillmore said. "So what's the difference between a problem and a predicament?" The mischievous teacher's smile returned to his face.

"A problem can be solved, but there is no solution for a predicament. You can deal with a problem but you have to live with a predicament. When you take this promise to heart, though, you don't whine or complain about either one. Deal with it or live with it, don't moan about it. And don't point fingers and blame other people. To me, this promise means that I accept full responsibility for my circumstances and my outcomes. I am where I am today because of choices I have made in the past, and no other reason. And I will be where I end up in the future because of choices I make from this point on, and no other reason. That is accepting responsibility for your life."

"I'm impressed," Fillmore said.

"I'm a Certified Values Coach Trainer," Jennifer replied. "I've put a lot of thought into these promises. I need to know what I'm talking about so I can do a good job teaching the course on The Twelve Core Action Values." Now she placed a finger on the third line of the certificate. "Being fully engaged means thinking like an owner and not just renting a spot on the organization chart." She ran a finger under the text on the certificate. "These are the eight essential characteristics of a culture of ownership. By signing the certificate we are promising ourselves to be committed to the mission, vision, and values of Midland Health; to be fully engaged in our work and with our coworkers; to be passionate about the work we do every day; to take initiative and do the right thing without waiting for someone else to give us permission or orders; to be good stewards of the organization's resources – including the time for which we are being paid to get work done; to promote a sense of belonging and a spirit of ownership in the organization; and to take pride in ourselves and the work we do, in our colleagues and our organization, and in the community we live in.""Very impressive," Fillmore said as he finished making a note in his steno pad. "But what if someone just wants to come to work and do the job and not feel like they have to do this whole ownership thing?"

Jennifer shrugged. "We still have a few people like that, but not too many. People who just want to be paid for coming to work but don't want to be expected to be emotionally positive, to be self empowered, and to get engaged probably aren't going to be very happy here."

Fillmore followed Jennifer along the corridor toward the last of the certificates. "New employees have their certificates added down here at the end." Jennifer pointed toward the empty space at the end of the long rows of signed certificates. "Hmm, that's strange," she said, tipping her head to one side. "These two weren't here this morning."

Fillmore put on his reading glasses and looked at the spot where the two most recently signed certificates had been mounted on the wall and read the names:

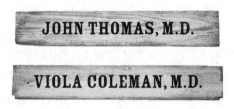

Fillmore ran his fingers across the two certificates. "Look how yellowed the paper is on these two. It looks like they've been here for a long time, and not just been posted since this morning."

Viola Coleman smiled and said, "They have been here for a long time." John Thomas nodded in agreement. Then they followed as Jennifer and the reporter continued down the hall toward the training room.

> PEOPLE WHO JUST WANT TO BE PAID FOR COMING TO WORK BUT DON'T WANT TO BE EXPECTED TO BE EMOTIONALLY POSITIVE, TO BE SELF EMPOWERED, AND TO GET ENGAGED PROBABLY AREN'T GOING TO BE VERY HAPPY HERE.

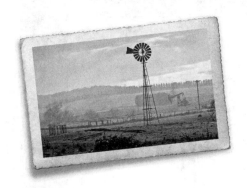

CHAPTER 8

Cindy Tinker was sitting alone in the Culture of Owner-ship training room contemplating the two wall-mounted displays with The Twelve Core Action Values course. She'd first become a Certified Values Coach Trainer because she loved Midland Memorial Hospital and wanted to be part of anything that would make the hospital a better place. In a thirty year career she'd gone from a starting job as a patient care assistant to now being a doctorally prepared clinical educator. *Where else would I have gotten that kind of support for my career?* she asked herself. And now she was in a position to repay the investment the hospital had made in her career by helping others make an investment in their lives. She didn't know that she was about to have four visitors, only two of whom she would ever know about.

Cindy and her team of Values Trainers would be teaching the course the following week for a group of new employees, including people from the two rural critical access hospitals that had just joined the Midland Health network and as part of that were able to send their people through the course. It

The Twelve Core Action Value
and the Cornerstones that Put Action into those Values

Laying a Solid Foundation

The first 6 Core Action Values help you develop strength of character.

1. Authenticity
Self Awareness
Self Mastery
Self Belief
Self Truth

2. Integrity
Honesty
Reliability
Humility
Stewardship

3. Awareness
Mindfulness
Objectivity
Empathy
Reflection

4. Courage
Confrontation
Transformation
Action
Connection

5. Perseverence
Preperation
Perspective
Toughness
Learning

6. Faith
Gratitude
Forgiveness
Love
Spirituality

The Twelve Core Action Value
and the Cornerstones that Put Action into those Values

Taking Effective Action

The second 6 Core Action Values catalyze action and inspire contribution.

7. Purpose
Aspiration
Intentionality
Selflessness
Balance

8. Vision
Attention
Imagination
Articulation
Belief

9. Focus
Target
Concentration
Speed
Momentum

10. Enthusiasm
Attitude
Energy
Curiosity
Humor

11. Service
Helpfulness
Charity
Compassion
Renewal

12. Leadership
Expectations
Example
Encouragement
Celebration

was the fourth time her team had taught the course and she was confident that they knew the material, but it was her own private ritual to sit alone in this room and reflect upon what she was going to say for the values she would be covering. Especially the stories from coworkers. She knew that for most participants the course was only theory until they heard about how people they actually knew and worked with were changing their lives as a result of having gone through it.

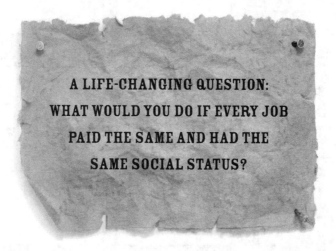

A LIFE-CHANGING QUESTION:
WHAT WOULD YOU DO IF EVERY JOB
PAID THE SAME AND HAD THE
SAME SOCIAL STATUS?

This time Cindy would be kicking off the course by teaching Core Action Value number one – Authenticity. For this one she was going to tell her own story. When she had taken the course to become a certified trainer, she'd been pulled up short by a question her instructor asked the class to think about: *What would you do if every job paid the same and had the same social status?* The question had brought back a flood of memories. She loved being a nurse, and was an excellent nurse – all her patients said so. But when she was growing up, she'd always wanted to be a teacher. She would actually set up classrooms in her back yard and teach classes to neighborhood kids. Taking the class, and asking herself that question, made her realize that her real calling – the work that would help her be her authentic best self – was to combine her love of nursing with her passion for teaching. The very next day she'd started working on applications for graduate school and had never looked back. *That question changed my life,* she whispered out loud, not realizing that Dr. John Thomas and Dr. Viola Coleman were standing in the back of the room.

"Honey," Viola Coleman said, knowing that Cindy would not hear her, "one way or another education will always change your life, and always for the better. And teaching is the way you take what you have learned and use it to help other people change their lives."

Cindy looked back toward the door but it was still closed and she could see no one else in the room. After her two fellow Values Trainers covered Integrity and Awareness, Core Action Values number two and three, Cindy would take over with Core Action Value #4, Courage. She still wasn't sure which story she wanted to tell to illustrate this value and its four cornerstones. The last time she'd taught the course she told the story of Ronnie Williamson, who after taking the values course had finally had the courage to finish the book he'd been putting off doing for many years, and was now a published author. And, he'd recently told her, was finding he needed even more courage to try and sell the book than he'd needed to write it.

But this time she was leaning toward telling the story of her good friend Jeanine Watson because it reflected the fourth cornerstone of the value – connection. Jeanine was an outstanding pediatric nurse, but not many people knew her because she was shy and introspective. In fact, some people thought of her as being downright unfriendly. That is, until in a one year period Jeanine lost her husband and was diagnosed with cancer. At first, Jeanine had tried to keep her problems to herself. "No one wants to carry my burdens for me," she'd told Cindy. But when word got out what she was going through, the people of Midland Health literally wrapped Jeanine into a big collective hug. She received financial support from the employee assistance fund, people donated paid time off so she would be able to pay her bills while going through treatment, and most important, Cindy thought, she'd been convinced to join the cancer support group that was sponsored by the Coleman Clinic.

"And that's what gave her the courage to face her challenges bravely," Cindy said aloud. "Maybe for the first time in her life she really felt connected to other people."

"Sorry, are we interrupting?" Cindy turned again and saw that Jennifer Scholander and a man she'd never seen before had come into the room.

Cindy jumped out of her chair. "Oh, hi Jennifer – I was just sitting in here talking with some of my invisible friends."

"If she only knew!" Viola Coleman said and John Thomas guffawed – wondering if he laughed loud enough he would break through the barrier that separated the two astral visitors from the corporeal beings in the room. But no one seemed to notice.

"Don't let us bother you," Jennifer said. "This is Harold Fillmore from *The Wall Street Journal*. He's writing a story about how Midland became recognized as the healthiest communities in Texas, and about how Midland Health has been honored for being one of the best places to work in the state."

Fillmore extended a hand. "Nice to meet you Cindy. Mind if we disturb you and your invisible friends for a minute with a few questions?"

"Not at all," Cindy replied, still a bit embarrassed at having been caught talking out loud to a room full of air.

Fillmore had pulled out his steno pad. He pointed to the two displays with The Twelve Core Action Values. "So I thought that Midland Health had three core values – Pioneer Spirit, Caring Heart, and Healing Mission." It was obvious that he was proud of himself for already knowing these by heart. "But this," and he waved with his hand "looks a whole lot more complicated. Are these more hospital values?"

"No sir," Cindy replied. "This is a course on personal values. If you look at the twelve values, and the four corner-stones for each value, you'll see that these are the values that inspire people to achieve their most important goals and become their best selves as people. From Authenticity, Core Action Value number one, through Leadership, Core Action Value number 12, these are values that – no matter what a person's religious belief or non-belief, their politics, their ethnic heritage or any other factor – we all want to live."

Cindy pointed to the yin-yang symbol on another wall. "This symbol reflects our appreciation of the interaction between personal values and organi-zational values. For Midland Health as an organization to really reflect a Pioneer Spirit, our people need to practice courage and perseverance – Core

Organizational Values

Personal Values

Action Values four and five. A caring heart at the organizational level requires individual employees who have faith – Core Action Value number six – and who are committed to service – Core Action Value number eleven. And for the organization to have a Healing Mission, we need individual employees who have a strong sense of purpose – Core Action Value number seven – and a shared vision for the future – Core Action Value number 8. Does that help?"

"Absolutely," Fillmore replied as he snapped photos of the values displays and the yin-yang symbol. Then he looked back at the values displays and asked, "So what are the words under each of the values?"

Cindy walked over to the display for the first six Core Action Values. "For each of the twelve values there are four cornerstones. These are the pillars that uphold that value – they are the personal expectations that put action into the value. And without action, values are just good intentions. So to work on becoming your authentic, meant-to-be best self – Core Action Value number one is Authenticity – requires these four things: self-awareness, self-mastery, self-belief, and self-truth. Those are the four cornerstones. Then for each cornerstone there are very practical techniques for working on that cornerstone. So, for example, one of the best ways to enhance self-awareness is by writing in a personal journal. As part of the course we give people a 360-Day Journal that challenges them with questions, quotes, and exercises to think about how you can do a better job of living these values. That's how the course works."

"Very impressive," Fillmore said as he scribbled in his steno pad.

Cindy nodded. "I also want to stress that these values aren't just about the work you do here for Midland Health. They apply to every dimension of our personal lives. I know that trying harder to incorporate these values into my own life has helped me become a better mother and a better person beyond being a better nurse and a better educator."

Dr. Coleman nodded appreciatively and said to Dr. Thomas, "When I worked here new employee orientation was about as exciting as watching a tumbleweed on a windless day. Oh my, how they would drone on about this policy and that procedure while the poor newbies struggled to stay awake. I don't imagine they're going to have any trouble keeping people awake by showing them how to be better parents and better people." Thomas nodded his agreement and said, "Yes, I think we tend to just assume that people know what their values are – but we all need periodic reminders about how to live those values."

Fillmore was about to put the steno pad back into his pocket when Cindy said, "One more thing. Like anything else in the world, people will get out of this course what they put into it. It can be life-changing or it can be a waste of time – that's a choice each individual will make. But I always remind people of this essential fact: the goals you achieve, the contribution you make, and the person you become will, more than any other single thing, be determined by the values that guide your decisions and your actions. That is the power of this course – it helps people do a better job of living the values that are essential for a good life."

Jennifer had been rocking back and forth on her toes with her arms crossed, the way she always did when she was thinking. "We actually see The Twelve Core Action Values course as a gift to our people that is also an investment in our organization. If people use this course to help them in their own personal lives and professional careers, it can't help but have a positive impact on patient satisfaction, employee morale, productivity, and every other aspect of what we do at Midland Health. And we have absolutely seen that happen."

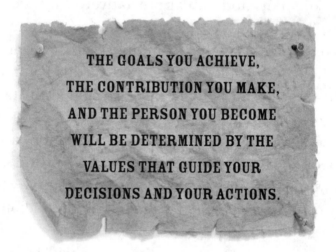

THE GOALS YOU ACHIEVE, THE CONTRIBUTION YOU MAKE, AND THE PERSON YOU BECOME WILL BE DETERMINED BY THE VALUES THAT GUIDE YOUR DECISIONS AND YOUR ACTIONS.

Fillmore had reopened his steno pad and was again taking notes. Cindy continued. "Anyone who takes to heart and acts upon Core Action Values one through eleven will become the sort of person who, by living his or her values, will influence and inspire other people to do the same. And that is the best definition I can think of for a leader: someone who inspires and influences others. You've heard the phrase Proceed Until Apprehended today."

Fillmore laughed. "I think those three words are going to start popping up in my dreams!"

Jennifer and Cindy both laughed as well, then Cindy said, "When we cover Core Action Value number twelve, Leadership, in the course we tell people to remember that you don't need a title to be a true leader. Management is a job description; leadership is a life decision. And it's not just being a leader here at work. It's being a leader in your community, in your church. It's inspiring your children to have big dreams and influencing them to have the work ethic that's required to make those dreams come true."

"If you want the secret of our success in just three words," Jennifer said, "those three words would be Proceed Until Apprehended. Midland never would have been recognized as the healthiest community in Texas, and Midland Health would never have been recognized as one of the best places to work in healthcare, if everyone waited for every decision to come down from above. To build a culture of ownership, and

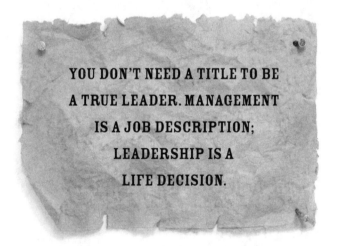

YOU DON'T NEED A TITLE TO BE
A TRUE LEADER. MANAGEMENT
IS A JOB DESCRIPTION;
LEADERSHIP IS A
LIFE DECISION.

to foster an empowered community, we needed leadership in every corner, not just in the corner offices. That's what The Twelve Core Action Values course here at Midland Health – and The Midland Year of Values project in the larger community – has helped us achieve. A community full of people who think and act like leaders – who are willing to Proceed Until Apprehended and do the right things."

Jennifer waited for Fillmore to finish making his notes then said, "We should leave Cindy and her invisible friends alone so they can continue their conversation – and we have more stops to make." Fillmore thanked Cindy for her time then followed Jennifer to the door.

"John," Viola Coleman said to Dr. Thomas, "I think it's time for Cindy's invisible friends to take their leaves as well. Let's let this young lady finish her contemplations in peace. I want to see where Jennifer is going to be taking this reporter next."

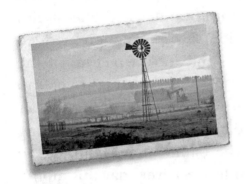

CHAPTER 9

"**S**o, where are we headed to first?" Fillmore slung his sports coat over his shoulder as he and Jennifer walked through the parking lot toward her car. They'd wrapped up their interviews at the main campus and were now setting out for a quick driving tour of some of the other facilities that were part of Midland Health and other partnering organizations before Jennifer dropped Fillmore off at the airport.

"We'll start with the Coleman Clinic, named for Dr. Viola Coleman – the woman whose bust you saw by the elevator on the sixth floor. They are a community health center that provides preventive and primary care regardless of any patient's ability to pay for the services."

Fillmore had just put on his sunglasses when he stopped short in front of one of the parking lot's lampposts. "What's that?" he asked, pointing to a large colorful banner emblazoned with the word PERSEVERANCE in big block letters, and in smaller print the words Preparation, Perspective, Toughness, and Learning.

"Remember when I mentioned Midland's Year of Values – when almost every business, church, government office, school, and other organization in town devoted one month to each of The Twelve Core Action Values?" Fillmore nodded then pulled out his cell phone and took a picture of the banner. Jennifer continued. "Well, during that year you saw these banners – one for each month – displayed all over the city. That went over so well that many of us, including Midland Health, have saved the banners and continue to put them up as ongoing reminders. So every day this month when I walk through this parking lot I'm reminded that to persevere toward achieving my goals I need to prepare myself for the inevitable challenges that will crop up, have a positive perspective when they do, face them with mental toughness, and learn the lessons that they bring. Those are the four cornerstones of Core Action Value number five, Perseverance."

"Wow," Fillmore said as he pocketed his cell phone. "You think about that every day?"

> THIS MIRACLE OF MIDLAND IS
> A STORY OF HOW AN ENTIRE
> COMMUNITY CAME TOGETHER WITH A
> COMMITMENT TO LIVE THEIR VALUES
> AND TAKE PRIDE OF OWNERSHIP
> IN THEIR ORGANIZATIONS.

"Actually twice a day – once going in and once coming out."

When Jennifer pulled into the parking lot of the Coleman Clinic with Fillmore in the passenger seat, Dr. John Thomas and Dr. Viola Coleman were already standing there, though of course the people in the car could not see them. Dr. Thomas looked at the sign over the door. "That's quite a tribute, Viola, having a clinic that serves the entire community named after you."

Coleman nodded. "I suppose so – they must have already used Kennedy and King to name more important things." Then she winked and smiled, and it was obvious how proud she was to have her legacy recognized in the naming of the clinic she had done so much to establish. The two physicians followed Scholander and Fillmore into the building.

Inside, the waiting room was packed with people of all ages and ethnicities. Some were clearly sick while others sat as if calmly waiting for a haircut appointment. "Now this is the sort of setting I remember," Coleman said with a smile. She rubbed her hands together as if she were ready to go to work and start seeing patients right away. Thomas shook his head in amazement. When he'd first moved to Midland, half the population of the city might have fit in this waiting room.

A man in a brown suitcoat came out from the registration area. "Good morning, Jennifer," he said as he shook her hand, then extended a hand to the reporter and said "and you must be Mr. Fillmore. I'm Lennie Phillips – I've been director here for almost two years. My predecessor got himself elected to the U.S. Congress. That's not a fate I would wish upon myself, but he's done some great things for healthcare here in West

Texas. Can I show you around, Mr. Fillmore, introduce you to some of our people?"

Fillmore smiled. "Just Harold. At The Journal there's only one 'mister' and he sits in a corner office that I only see about twice a year. So can you give me a few examples of the sorts of things you've done to promote better health in Midland?"

"We do a lot of a lot of things," Phillips said, "from dental to mental, from babies to old folks, we have the busiest community health center in West Texas. And we're expanding in directions that wouldn't even have been imaginable five or six years ago. Much more emphasis today on health promotion and disease prevention – and we're seeing some remarkable successes on that front."

Phillips pointed to a shiny new plaque on the wall. "Lots of them. We've received national recognition for the way we're working with law enforcement and employers to reduce domestic violence..."

"Yeah," Fillmore interrupted, "I just saw the news about the award you received last month – congratulations."

"Thanks," Phillips replied. "That was a top priority – still is. I'm also proud of the way we've partnered with the schools to bring more health education and healthy lifestyle training into the educational process. And we're working with the city to establish more bike lanes and hiking trails. But my favorite activities are the hiking trips we take our kids on. Next month I'll be going on one to Big Bend National Park."

"So," Fillmore said, "your clinic has really been on the front lines with the changes we've seen in the healthcare system over the past decade. What are some of the ways you've responded?"

"Great question. Probably the most important is the way we've reached out to the community. We know we can't just sit in the clinic waiting for sick people to come to us – we need to reach out and help make sure that they don't need to come to us. Not that we don't love them – we do! – we just would rather see them out and about doing good work than…" and he nodded in the direction of people crowded into the waiting room, "and not in here waiting for us to treat their illnesses."

Fillmore had pulled out his steno pad and was taking notes. "What are some of the ways you do that?"

"Sure," Phillips replied. "We've worked with the city to help them establish more bike lanes and hiking trails, but they don't do much good for kids who don't have bikes or hiking shoes, so we've also set up a philanthropic program to get bikes and helmets for kids who couldn't otherwise afford them – and give them lessons on how to safely use them. I'll tell you more as we walk around, but since I know you have a plane to catch let's take a quick tour. We are very proud of the Coleman Clinic."

"I'm very proud of the people who work in the Coleman Clinic," Dr. Coleman said with conviction, though of course only Dr. Thomas could hear her.

Phillips walked them through their dental clinic, the radiology suite, and the adult clinic. "We're very proud of our new addition," he said, pointing to a door labeled Alternative Therapies. "We can't go back there now because there are patients, but we are one of the first community health clinics in the nation to have comprehensively embraced alternative therapies for health and healing. We have three massage therapists, an acupuncturist, and specialists in healing touch and Reiki on our staff. Most places these services are limited to upscale white collar neighborhoods – we're proud to be able to offer them to everyone who can benefit, regardless of their financial status."

Phillips tapped a picture frame mounted on a table in the main intersection of the clinic. "This is Dr. Viola Coleman, for whom our clinic was named. I never met her, but from everything I hear she was a real force of nature."

Fillmore chuckled. "That's not the first time I've heard her described like that today." Then he looked more closely at Phillips' hand. "I see you are wearing one of those colored Pledge bracelets I've seen all over the hospital. Are you doing that here too?"

Phillips gave his wristband a snap. "Every day. Several times a day a group will meet right here by Dr. Coleman's picture and together say that day's promise. But we also share The Self Empowerment Pledge with our patients. More than half of the problems we see could be prevented if people would take better care of themselves, and that's what these promises are – a commitment to take better care of oneself."

Fillmore pursed his lips skeptically. "You know, Lennie, at least since King Solomon sat down to write the Book of Proverbs wise men and motivational speakers have been telling us that we need to take better care of ourselves but you don't see a whole lot of evidence that's it's working very well. What makes this different?"

Phillips rubbed his chin thoughtfully. He didn't hear Dr. Coleman mutter to Dr. Thomas, "I'm going to be interested to hear what he has to say about this one." Then he said, "Let me tell you a story. One day last year a woman stopped by my office. She looked familiar but for the life of me I couldn't place her. You want to know why? Since the last time I'd seen her she'd lost more than a hundred pounds, she'd quit smoking, and she was exercising every day. You know how she did it?"

Fillmore shrugged. Phillips continued. "When I asked her she just said Monday, Tuesday, and Wednesday. Then she recited those three promises on Responsibility, Accountability, and Determination from memory – and showed me that she was wearing all three of those wristbands. She said that it wasn't until she accepted personal responsibility for her health, held herself accountable for the results she achieved, and was determined to do the work that she started to lose weight and regain her health."

Fillmore was writing in his steno pad. "That is pretty impressive. I need to catch a plane today but do you think you could arrange for me to speak with her by phone later this week?"

Phillips nodded toward Jennifer. "I'm sure Jennifer can – Lestelle now volunteers at the hospital several days a week." Jennifer made a note of Lestelle's name and agreed to make the connection.

They were now walking into the pediatric clinic. In between the Disney and Dr. Seuss characters on the wall Fillmore saw a big smiling pickle. "So you've gotten on the pickle band-wagon too, I see," he said, looking at Phillips.

"You bet," Phillips replied. "At first it was just something we were doing for our staff, but when patients we started including them as well. And now every patient gets a one page instruction sheet – I'll make sure you get one before you leave – on how to turn their home into a PFZ, a Pickle-Free Zone."

Fillmore laughed. "I'm trying to imagine the reaction of my wife and kids if I came home and declared our house was going to be a Pickle-Free Zone – and I assume I'd have to tell them it was going to cost them a quarter every time they would whine or complain?"

"That's the idea," Phillips said with a smile. "But here's the deal. At first almost no one takes this seriously. But then they start hearing from neighbors, or from the person sitting next to them in the waiting room, what a difference it's making. And – just as it has over at Midland Memorial Hospital – The Pickle Challenge has really taken on a life of its own among our people. And I'll tell you – one of the places where the wristbands and the pickle have been most powerful is in some of the support groups we sponsor. You know, these folks are dealing with some pretty serious problems. We might not be able to make their cancer go away, cure them of their addictions, or make lost loved ones come back, but we can help them have the strength to find the blessings in their lives and to help make a difference in the lives of other people. That's often the real miracle – not a magical cure but rather a spiritual healing."

Fillmore pursed his lips again. "It's my job to be skeptical, but I have to tell you that this all sounds a bit Pollyanna to me."

"Oh, indeed," Phillips replied with a laugh, "it certainly is. But if you would actually go read the story Pollyanna you'd see that she was an incredibly kind and courageous young woman who, despite her own personal tragedies, helped bring healing to a community that was broken and in a great deal of pain. So I take being called Pollyanna as a great compliment – and see her story as a great metaphor for what we are called to do."

On their way to the airport, Jennifer singled out some of the other activities in which Midland Health had been involved. She pointed to an obviously new three-story building and said "That is the new Midland Health Center for the Patient Experience. They are doing cutting edge research on clinical quality, creating a safer healthcare environment, and assuring a great patient experience." On the next block she pointed to a big sign that read Midland Fit – Midland Strong. "That is the new community health and fitness center. It's a partnership between Midland Health, the Coleman Clinic, the local YMCA, and was built with substantial philanthropic support from the community. And it's now financially self-sustaining through programs and memberships. We are very proud of these two new developments."

"I can see that," Fillmore said as he took pictures through the car window.

At the airport Jennifer helped Fillmore retrieve his bag from the trunk then gave him a hug. "West Texas friendly," she said with a dimpled smile. "Hugs are better than handshakes."

Fillmore stood in the West Texas sunshine for a long while before heading into the airport to catch his flight back to New York City. There really was something special going on out here in the prairies of West Texas.

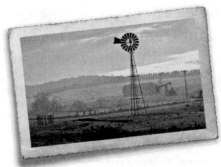

CHAPTER 10

When Harold Fillmore placed his cell phone over the scanner to board his flight from Dallas to New York City the machine beeped three times and spit out a little slip of paper. "Well, Mr. Fillmore, it's your lucky day," the gate agent said as she handed him the paper. "You've been upgraded to first class."

Fillmore stowed his bag in the overhead and nestled into seat 3A. When the flight attendant came by he ordered black coffee then pulled the steno pad, which was now almost completely filled with notes, from his pocket. He took being upgraded to first class – something that had never happened in more than a quarter-century of reporting – to be an omen that his article would indeed grace the front page of *The Wall Street Journal.* He'd sketched out a first draft of "The Miracle of Midland" while waiting for his flight. That would be, he'd decided, the title of the article.

He pulled a yellow pad from his backpack, took a sip of coffee, and started to write.

"There were seven key success factors underlying this Miracle of Midland," he wrote. "Taken together, these seven factors constitute a formula for successful culture change and can be used by any organization, any community, or for that matter any family to foster a more positive cultural environment. These seven factors are:"

Key Success Factor #1 – Vision

It began with an understanding at Midland Health that they had to devote as much time and energy to defining their Invisible Architecture of core values, organizational culture, and workplace attitude as they had put into designing their beautiful physical facilities. They actually created a Cultural Blueprint that established common expectations regarding attitudes and behaviors that would reflect the Invisible Architecture they had designed.

Key Success Factor #2 – Courage

They had the courage to enforce those higher expectations. They defined zero tolerance behaviors – what they call ZTBs – and began to hold one another to a higher standard of behavior. For this reporter, the biggest surprise came in hearing story after story about how people had taken what started as a workplace initiative home with them and worked to create a more positive family culture on the home front. This highlights the key point that culture does not change unless and until people change, and people will make sustained personal changes only to the extent that they see an important personal benefit to doing so.

Key Success Factor #3 – Values

They understood the power of values as a foundation for everything else. When Midland Health defined its core values of Pioneer Spirit, Caring Heart, and Healing Mission – and then shared the course on The Twelve Core Action Values with all of its employees – they laid the foundation for sweeping cultural changes that were quickly reflected in increased employee engagement, higher patient satisfaction, greater productivity, and for being recognized as a great place to work. And at a personal level, when people made a commitment to living their personal values they were more successful at quitting smoking, losing weight, eating right, getting exercise, and all-in-all being happier and healthier individuals.

Key Success Factor #4 – Catalytic Events

They employed catalytic events to give an exclamation point to the culture change process. In this reporter's eyes, The Pickle Challenge for Charity was the initial spark that transformed what could have been seen as just another management program into an organization-wide movement across Midland Health. And when Midland Health led the *Midland's Year of Values* project in which the entire city made a one-year commitment to The Twelve Core Action Values, focusing on one value each month for a year, it galvanized the entire community.

Key Success Factor #5 – Grassroots Commitment

While the initiative started from the top, what really gave momentum to this movement – and it really does feel like a movement, not a program – was what I think of as 360-degree leadership. Over and over I heard the phrase "Proceed Until Apprehended" often followed by stories about how people had taken the initiative to go above and beyond the call of duty. That commitment to leadership not just in the corner office but in every corner of the organization was, I believe, the essential ingredient to making a culture of ownership part of the Midland Health cultural DNA.

Key Success Factor #6 – Perseverance

Although there were some rough spots along the way, including significant external challenges related to health-care reform and reimbursement cuts, they never allowed this effort to degenerate into just another program of the month. It was my sense that somewhere between the second and third years of their commitment to a culture of ownership that they hit a critical mass where they had achieved suffi-cient forward momentum that nothing would cause them to backslide. This was most evident, I thought, in the number of stories I heard about employees being willing to work short-staffed rather than to allow a warm body with a bad attitude to come in and pollute their culture.

Key Success Factor #7 — Community Focus

Ultimately, the culture of any organization is a subset of the culture of the broader community. This reporter has seen many organizational culture initiatives backslide and eventually fail because, as well-meaning as they were, when people left work they'd be dragged down by a more negative community culture, and in some cases a more negative family culture. When Midland Health convinced the entire community – businesses, educational institutions, government agencies, churches, social services organizations, and the media – to all commit to The Year of Values, it was as if they flipped a cultural switch. Instead of swimming against a current of cultural negativity they began to surf a wave of cultural positivity. And as each individual entity began to see the improvements in their own results, it sparked a self-perpetuating cycle. A commitment to values and a culture of ownership is becoming part of the cultural DNA of the entire community.

Fillmore was surprised to hear the flight attendant giving the final instructions before landing at LaGuardia. He'd been so absorbed in his writing he had completely lost track of time. He drained his last cup of coffee and handed the empty cup to the flight attendant. He looked out the window at the city below. Then he wrote what would be the last few sentences of his article.

The Making of a Miracle

It takes a special eye to appreciate the beauty of West Texas. Midland has no mountain vistas on the horizon, and the city is not blessed with a beautiful river or deep green lakes. You won't hear gentle breezes rustling through the branches of pine forests – you'll see strong winds whipping tumbleweeds across the prairies. But Midland has something that in its own way is just as beautiful. They call it West Texas Friendly, and you feel it the moment you hit the city. There is indeed something special happening out there on the prairies. This Miracle of Midland is a story of how an entire community came together with a commitment to live their values and to take pride of ownership in their organizations. And with the formula I've just described, they've shown us how we can all accomplish that same miracle where we work and where we live.

Harold Fillmore took one last look at what he had just written. He didn't see the two people looking over his shoulder. "Well, Viola," Dr. John Thomas said to the woman that only he could see, "what do you think?"

Dr. Viola Coleman smiled. "I think we can go home now – the work we started is in good hands."

EPILOG

The year was 2041. A soft breeze blew in from the west as Jennifer Scholander walked out onto the roof of the Scharbauer Tower. Stars beyond counting had claimed their places in a moonless sky as the last traces of sunset faded on the horizon. There had been a lovely celebration earlier in the evening. This morning Jennifer had been CEO of Midland Health, a position she'd held for the previous seven years. After this evening's retirement party she was Jennifer Scholander, private citizen. Tomorrow she would turn in her name badge and her keys so tonight would be the last time she would ever be able to stand alone on the roof, which over the years had become her favorite place to think.

As she looked out over a city that had transformed itself from an oil town at the beginning of the century to the most diversified business hub in West Texas now, she thought back on the history of the hospital and imagined Dr. John Thomas, the man who more than a century earlier had founded what became Midland Memorial Hospital on the second floor of a hotel, standing there with her in his boots and cowboy hat. *The Pioneer Spirit that you instilled in your little hospital is alive and well at Midland Health, Dr. Thomas.* That's what she would have said to the good doctor had he actually been there. Over the past quarter century Midland Memorial Hospital had grown from a very ordinary small town hospital that had to send the sickest and most severely injured patients to distant cities for care, into Midland Health – a comprehensive medical center offering a full range of services for a growing city.

In the distance Scholander heard a helicopter approaching from the north. When she'd first started at Midland Health as a staff nurse, an approaching helicopter often meant that a Midlander was about to be transported to Lubbock or Dallas for advanced care. Today it almost always meant that EMS was bringing a very sick or very seriously injured patient to MMH for advanced care. The Pioneer Spirit had become so deeply ingrained into the DNA of the organization that hardly a day went by that Scholander hadn't been asked to consider a new service or program. Tomorrow, she thought, all of those proposals will land on the desk of her successor.

Scholander watched the helicopter land and the crew unload an isolette incubator. At one time that baby, and the baby's parents, would have had to go to a faraway city; today they could receive the most advanced and sophisticated care right here in the neonatal intensive care unit of Midland Memorial Hospital. And if that baby's grandparents needed skilled care, the hospital had a pioneering Acute Care for the Elderly unit. From pregnancy to end of life, Midland Health had been a pioneer in advancing healthcare for the people of West Texas and beyond.

Looking out over the city, Scholander thought about Dr. Viola Coleman. She'd heard stories about how Coleman would come in at all hours, making rounds in a house coat and slippers. Dr. Coleman truly had represented the Caring

Heart value of Midland Health, and that value was now woven deeply into the cultural fabric of the organization. Earlier in the week Scholander had attended a recognition ceremony for the latest nurse to receive a DAISY Award. She had received more than a dozen letters from patients wanting to commend their caregivers, had stopped by the Pharmacy to congratulate an employee on the occasion of her 40th anniversary working at the hospital, and had heard about how a long-time employee in Nutrition Services recently diagnosed with cancer was receiving an outpouring of emotional support from coworkers and financial support from the catastrophic employee assistance program. The commitment to a caring heart lived on across the entire Midland Health system.

Of all the things she was most proud of, Scholander thought to herself, that was at the top of the list: the way Midland Health truly was a caring organization. When Midland Health had been recognized by a national business magazine as being one of the hundred best places to work in America, and each year since had moved up in the rankings, more than anything it was because of the caring heart of the people who worked there. That caring spirit was reflected from the moment someone pulled up to the front door for valet parking, through the smiles of passersby in the hallways, to the care they received in the hospital, and on through the health promotion services that Midland Health provided to the community.

Scholander watched a plane circling for a landing at the Midland airport. It was, she knew, the last flight in from Dallas. She also knew that one of the passengers was a consultant on community health promotion who'd been working with the hospital for the past several years. She thought back on one of the last conversations she'd had with the previous CEO about expanding the Healing Mission of Midland Health beyond the walls of the hospital to include a greater focus on health promotion and disease prevention.

Through a combination of new services and partnerships with existing organizations, Midland Health had developed a comprehensive community health plan – and it was paying off. Midland had long ago been recognized as being one of the healthiest communities in the state of Texas, and more recently a reporter from *Texas Monthly* had been in town interviewing people for an article on how the city had been able to establish health promotion as a priority in the business sector, in the school system, and in families across the community.

Pioneer Spirit, Caring Heart, Healing Mission. From the beginning those three values had defined Midland Memorial Hospital, and in the years to come they would guide the priorities of Midland Health. And they would inspire the three thousand people who worked for the organization – not just in their work, but also at home in their personal and family lives. The nighttime chill of the desert was beginning to set in. Scholander had to remind herself that, for the first time in many years, she did not need to stop by the office to pick up a briefcase full of work on her way out. Tomorrow she was going to the beach.

THE END

APPENDIX 1

*Chronology of Key Events in the History of
Midland Memorial Hospital*

1944 In December, the Midland Chamber of Commerce
appointed a hospital committee to investigate and make
recommendations about the possibility of building a
community-owned hospital.

1945 The Chamber of Commerce's committee recom-
mended that a charitable non-profit corporation, to be
called Midland Memorial Foundation, be formed to solicit
contributions for the purpose of building and operating a
hospital. Twenty-five Midland citizens were selected to serve
on what is now the Board of Governors. By 1946, they had
raised only $260,000 for building a hospital. In 1947 they
launched an all-out drive and raised more than $750,000.
Matched by $400,000 in a government grant and 7 acres
of land donated by Mr. and Mrs. E. P. Cowden and Mr. and

Mrs. Clinton M. Dunagan, the Governors believed they had raised more than enough.

1948 Ground was broken for the hospital building.

1950 Midland Memorial Hospital, a four-story 75-bed facility, opened on July 11. Total cost: $1,125,000.

1955 $150,000 was raised to pay off outstanding obligations. The Midland County Commissioners Court and Midland City Council entered into long-term leases that made the financing of a new wing possible, coupled with another grant from the federal government.

1958 An $800,000 east wing expansion brought the total beds to 150.

1963 The 4th floor of the east wing was added to house surgery, a recovery room and a 9-bed Intensive Care Unit. Bed capacity increased to 178. The original part of the Hospital was air conditioned.

1966 The parking lot was paved.

1973 Phase I of a two-phase expansion (70,000 square feet) on the west end of the Hospital was completed, housing Surgery, Recovery, Anesthesia, Labor and Delivery, Radiology, Emergency Room, Purchasing, Central Services, Pharmacy, Cafeteria, Kitchen and Medical Records. Cost: $3.7 million.

1977 The Hospital District was formed and a $10 million expansion program was begun, financed by the only general obligation bond issue in the Hospital's history. This bond was paid off in 1997.

1979 Phase II of the expansion was completed, adding a new Maternity Wing and Critical Care and Post-Critical Care Units, and relocating the Cardiopulmonary Department.

Private bathrooms were added to the 1950s' building by placing the plumbing on the outside of the building and covering it with a stucco façade. Total beds: 195.

1986 A 3rd and 4th floor were added to the west expansion providing additional medical-surgical beds and a new obstetrics floor. New business offices, admitting, lobby and staff offices were completed. $15.1 million project. 272 beds.

1994 The north expansion changed the face of the Hospital and added almost 100,000 square feet for surgical facilities and support services, including the Emergency Department, Laboratory and the Testing and Diagnostic Center.

2001 Westwood Hospital was acquired. Labor and Delivery, Postpartum, Nursery and Pediatrics were consolidated at the renamed West Campus. The West Campus also included Outpatient Surgery, Imaging, Lab and its own Emergency Department.

2007 The new Medical Office Building opened on the north side of the Main Campus. This 88,000 square foot facility was financed in part by $6.5 million in private donations, and is the first high-quality medical office space built on the Main Campus in over 30 years. It houses a variety of physicians' offices, including Texas Oncology and Permian

Cardiology Associates, along with the Hospital's outpatient imaging center (Diagnostic Imaging Associates, or DIA).

2008 Campaign for Tomorrow begins to raise funds for new hospital tower with foundational contribution by Clarence Scharbauer Jr.

2009 Successful $115 million bond election.

2010 New patient tower groundbreaking with topping out ceremony in May of 2011.

2011 MMH is recognized as an ANCC Pathway to Excellence® organization for having a positive practice environment.

2012 Medical Office Building named for Nadine and Tom Craddick in honor of their dedicated service to healthcare in West Texas.

2012 Grand opening of the Dorothy and Clarence Scharbauer Jr. Patient Tower.

2013 Final stage of construction complete including Emergency Department, CT scanning, and conference center.

2014 MMH is recognized a second time as an ANCC Pathway to Excellence® organization.

2014 Launch of the Values and Culture Project and training of the inaugural corps of 40 Certified Values Coach Trainers.

A lot more will be added between now and 2041!

If we each do our part, we will change
our lives for the better.

If we all do our parts, we will change
our organizations for the better.

And in changing our organizations,
we can change our world for the better.

From *The Florence Prescription*

NOTES

NOTES

NOTES

NOTES